Metabolic Restoration

Metabolic Restoration

Returning to the Foundations of Health

Vanessa Menanteau, DNP, FNP, CNM

Metabolic Restoration

Returning to the Foundations of Health

First Edition, 2026
Interior Version 1.1 – August 2026

ISBN: 979-8-9968450-0-2

Published by Pura Vida Publishing
An imprint of Nutricion Pura Vida LLC

Cover Design and Interior Layout by Vanessa Menanteau

Printed in the United States of America

Disclaimer

The information presented in this book is intended for educational and informational purposes only. It is not intended to diagnose, treat, cure, or prevent any disease and should not be considered medical advice.

The content of this book is not a substitute for individualized medical care, diagnosis, or treatment provided by a qualified healthcare professional. Always consult your physician or other qualified healthcare provider regarding questions about your health, medical conditions, medications, supplements, or treatment plans.

Never disregard professional medical advice or delay seeking medical care because of something you have read in this book. The author and publisher assume no responsibility for any adverse effects or consequences resulting from the use of the information contained herein.

Table of Contents

To Those Who Shaped My Journey

Before these pages became a book, they were conversations, patients, questions, lessons, meals, friendships, motherhood, healing experiences, and many moments that helped define the way I see life, health, and human beings. There are countless people whose influence lives within these chapters, whether they realize it or not. This is for them.

To My Patients

Thank you for trusting me with your stories, your fears, your symptoms, your hopes, and your healing journeys. Medicine has taught me that people are not simply lab values, diagnoses, or protocols. Behind every appointment is someone trying to feel better, understand their body, and reclaim a sense of vitality in a world that often leaves people disconnected from themselves.

Some of you came to me exhausted, inflamed, discouraged, or unheard. Yet you remained open. You listened, you learned, you tried new things, and little by little, you transformed your health and your lives. Your courage, discipline, vulnerability, and trust have taught me far more than you know. This book was not written only from research or education. It was written through years of interactions with people like you. Thank you for allowing me to walk beside you.

To My Friends

Thank you for listening to years of ideas, reflections, voice messages, breakthroughs, frustrations, dreams, and reinventions. Some of you not only listened but courageously transformed your own lives. You became healthier, stronger, more aware, and more connected to yourselves because you were willing to question old habits and try something different. Watching those transformations has been profoundly inspiring to me.

Others may not have been ready to make big changes, and that is perfectly okay. Your love, respect, curiosity, encouragement, and belief in what I was building still mean more than you know. Every chat, every question, every shared meal, every moment of laughter and honesty helped shape the woman writing these pages.

And to a few extraordinary friends and colleagues who significantly influenced the way I think, practice, and dream, thank you! A special thank you to my friend and business partner, Dr. Oscar Aguilar, whose trust in me, belief in my vision, and respect for the way I practice medicine became an important part of this chapter of my life. Long before we built something together professionally, he was someone I deeply admired and trusted clinically. His friendship, insight, and encouragement helped expand what I believed was possible. Thank you for witnessing my evolution while allowing me to witness yours.

A very special thank you to my dear friend, Sandy. Her friendship, unwavering support, and contagious enthusiasm have been a priceless part of this journey. From our mountain walks, where so many ideas first came to life, to being one of this book's very first readers, she shared every step of this adventure with genuine excitement and joy. Thank you for celebrating this dream with me.

To My Parents and Grandparents

To my family, thank you for giving me such a beautiful foundation from which to begin life. Long before I understood nutrition, wellness, or medicine professionally, I was already living inside many of those values at home. Food was never treated as an afterthought. It was thoughtful, intentional, balanced, and intimately connected to well-being. Because of you, I grew up understanding that nourishment mattered. The impact of that gift has reached far beyond what you may ever fully realize. The way you cared for your bodies and the importance you placed on quality, health, and discipline became part of the fabric of who I am today.

Even across oceans, countries, careers, and different stages of life, your support has remained steady. And one of the things I cherish most is that you truly listened. You remained open to my evolving perspectives, trusted many of the things I was learning along the way, and allowed me to share my passion for health not only as your daughter or granddaughter but also as a healthcare provider.

Our family shapes us in visible and invisible ways. Some through softness, some through challenges, expectations, or through example. Looking back now, I can see how strongly all of it contributed to the woman I became. And while no family story is ever perfectly simple, I carry profound gratitude for the values, strength, resilience, and love that emerged from ours. Thank you for helping shape a life rooted in curiosity, growth, intention, and care.

To My Children

To my children, thank you for being some of my greatest teachers. Motherhood gave deeper meaning to everything I believed about nourishment, health, love, and intentional living. Raising you encouraged me to think differently, to question deeply, and to make choices with long-term well-being in mind.

I know there were moments when the way we lived or the foods I chose for our home may have felt different from what many of your friends experienced. You may not always have understood why I cared so much about what went into your bodies, your minds, and your environment. But every choice came from love. My greatest hope was to give you the strongest foundation possible — physically, emotionally, and spiritually — so you could move through life with health, resilience, and awareness.

Watching the incredible humans you have become fills me with more pride than words could ever express. And one day, I hope you will fully understand that so much of what I did, I did because I loved you fiercely.

Foreword

There are books that inform. There are books that inspire. And then, rarely, there are books that do both — books that arrive at exactly the right moment in history, written by exactly the right person, and manage to give a confused and suffering public something they have been searching for: Clarity, compassion, and a path forward. *Metabolic Restoration: Returning to the Foundations of Health* is precisely that kind of book. And I say that not as a courtesy, but as a physician who has spent decades watching the very crisis this book addresses unfold — one patient, one diagnosis, one missed opportunity at a time.

I have had the privilege of knowing Dr. Vanessa Menanteau for about six years. In that time, I have come to understand that she is not simply a clinician — she is a scholar, a healer, and a deeply determined advocate for a kind of medicine that most health systems have yet to find the courage to embrace. Her training as a Doctor of Nursing Practice, a Family Nurse Practitioner, and a Certified Nurse-Midwife already places her at the intersection of multiple dimensions of human health. But what distinguishes Dr. Menanteau is not her credentials. It is the way she sees people. With uncommon depth, she looks past symptoms and diagnoses to find the human being underneath — exhausted, often unheard, searching for answers that a fifteen-minute appointment can almost never provide.

My own journey through medicine has taken me from internal medicine to interventional cardiology, nuclear cardiology, and advanced cardiac imaging, and in more recent years into the fields of obesity medicine, metabolic medicine, hormone replacement therapy, nutrition, and public health. I founded Texas Integrative Medicine and Cardiology in El Paso, Texas, with a singular conviction: That the future of health lies not in more procedures, but in deeper prevention. I have also had the honor of contributing to metabolic health policy work at an international level, including the design of programs aimed at reversing the catastrophic burden of metabolic and cardiovascular disease in populations where these conditions have reached crisis proportions. In each of these experiences, one truth has repeated itself with relentless consistency: We are not suffering from a lack of medications. We are suffering from a profound disconnection from the foundations of health.

That is the crisis Dr. Menanteau names with both scientific precision and extraordinary compassion in this book. She does not shy away from difficult truths. She writes honestly about a healthcare system that was trained to wait for disease rather than preserve health, about food environments designed to overwhelm biology, about nervous systems that never fully rest, and about a culture that has normalized suffering to such a degree that people no longer recognize how unwell they have become. These are not comfortable observations. But they are accurate ones, and they are offered not to condemn, but to liberate.

What makes *Metabolic Restoration* exceptional is not any single chapter, though each one is rich with evidence, insight, and practical wisdom. What makes it exceptional is its architecture of understanding. Dr. Menanteau builds the reader's awareness systematically and gently, moving from the environmental forces shaping our biology to the physiological mechanisms being disrupted, and ultimately to a structured, compassionate, and evidence-informed program for restoration. She covers metabolism, insulin resistance, the truth about sugar, the transformative power of muscle, the role of sleep, the burden of toxin exposure, and the underappreciated spiritual dimension of health — all with a voice that never lectures, never condescends, and never loses sight of the human being she is trying to help.

The 28-Day Metabolic Restoration program at the heart of this book is not a fad. It is not a shortcut. It is a clinically thoughtful, physiologically sound framework for returning the body to conditions under which it was designed to thrive. As a physician who has guided countless patients through metabolic transformation — and who has seen firsthand how profoundly the body responds when given the right inputs consistently — I can affirm that the principles Dr. Menanteau presents here are grounded in the best available science and in deep clinical experience. They work. Not because they promise the impossible, but because they respect the remarkable intelligence of human physiology.

The metabolic crisis is not a local problem. It is a global one. Communities across the United States and far beyond our borders are facing epidemic rates of obesity, type 2 diabetes, cardiovascular disease, and chronic inflammation — conditions that are not inevitable, but that have been cultivated by modern environments and reinforced by systems of care that arrive too late. If we are to meaningfully bend those curves, it will require exactly what Dr. Menanteau offers here: Education that is honest, accessible, and grounded in both science and humanity. Books like this one are not supplementary to medicine. They are, in many ways, its most important frontier.

I am honored to introduce this work to you. Whether you are a patient searching for answers, a clinician seeking a resource you can confidently share, an educator committed to health literacy, or simply a person who has sensed for a long time that something in the way we live is not working — this book was written for you. Read it with openness. Trust what it asks of you. And know that the body you are living in is far more capable of restoration than you may have been led to believe.

Oscar M. Aguilar, MD, MPH, FACP, FAHA
Internal Medicine | Cardiology | Interventional Cardiology | Longevity Medicine
Founder, Texas Integrative Medicine and Cardiology, El Paso, Texas

METABOLIC
— RESTORATION —

Join the Free:

Metabolic Restoration Community

Why I Wrote This Book

Over the past few years, I have had the privilege of spending time in a world that is helping shape the future of medicine. It is a space filled with brilliant colleagues who are scientists, physicians, innovators, and entrepreneurs, and are working to better understand aging, longevity, and optimal wellness. Conversations often focus on advanced diagnostics, biological age, regenerative medicine, genomics, and the possibility of living longer than we ever imagined.

My other world is real life, where most people live. It is the world of individuals who are just trying to make it through the day. The contrast between those two worlds is striking. While the longevity community discusses how to extend life, most people are still struggling to build the foundations of health.

And that is why I wrote this book. Because before we can have meaningful conversations about living beyond 120, we need to help more people feel well at 40, 50, and beyond. We need to make the principles of health understandable, practical, and accessible to everyone. The path to extraordinary longevity begins with ordinary health.

Before You Begin

Before you turn the page and begin reading the introduction, I want to ask you to do something simple. Grab a pen or a pencil and turn to Appendix A. There, you will find the Pre-Program Metabolic Restoration Symptom Assessment. I encourage you to complete it honestly, based on how you truly feel right now, not how you think you "should" feel or how you hope to feel someday. Do not overthink your answers. Simply notice.

A notable aspect of human nature is how quickly we adapt to the way we feel. People often stop questioning the small ways they may no longer feel fully well because those sensations slowly become familiar. Certain sensations begin to feel so typical that they fade into the background of everyday life. That is part of the reason I want you to begin there. Not to judge or to label yourself. Only to create awareness.

At the end of this book, you will return to the back and complete the Post-Program Metabolic Restoration Symptom Assessment (Appendix B). My hope is that you begin observing yourself, your body, and your daily patterns with greater clarity than before.

And while you move through these pages, I want to encourage you to truly use this book. Underline sentences that resonate with you. Circle ideas that surprise you. Fold pages that you know you will want to revisit later. Write question marks besides concepts you have never considered before. Highlight passages that feel like they put words to something you have sensed intuitively for a long time but never fully understood. Let the book become interactive. Let it become personal.

Because sometimes a single idea, encountered at the right moment, can begin to change the direction of someone's life. Some sections of this book may resonate immediately. Others may challenge assumptions you have carried for years. Certain ideas may feel exciting, while others may require time to settle more completely before their meaning fully unfolds. That is perfectly okay. You do not need to absorb everything at once. This is not a race. It is an exploration.

So, before we begin, take a breath. Open Appendix A and answer honestly. And then turn to the next page and start reading with curiosity.

Introduction

Long before I practiced medicine, something about the way health was being approached never fully made sense to me. I grew up in Spain in a household where food was still recognizable, meals were cooked, and many of the habits people now call "wellness" were part of everyday life. At the time, I did not think of those things as extraordinary. They felt normal.

Years later, after moving to the United States, I remember reading one of Andrew Weil's books in the early 2000s and feeling as though a new door had opened. I still remember standing in front of my kitchen pantry reading ingredient labels differently for the first time. I remember learning about partially hydrogenated oils and discovering they were hiding in foods people consumed every day without thinking twice. I remember cleaning out my pantry and refrigerator afterward and feeling some sense of control over what I was feeding my family. What struck me most was the realization that everyday choices shape physiology far more than most of us realize.

Once I stepped into healthcare, I began to notice that people usually waited until their bodies became loud before paying attention to them. Symptoms were normalized, as were chronic illnesses. At the same time, science was beginning to reveal something profoundly hopeful: The body is far more dynamic, adaptable, and responsive than we once believed.

This book is about awareness, about learning to recognize the conversations happening inside the body long before a crisis arrives. It is about nourishment, metabolism, sleep, stress, muscle, longevity, prevention, and the extraordinary way physiology responds when we begin caring for ourselves more intentionally and consistently.

But beneath all of those topics lies something even deeper. This book is ultimately about our relationship with ourselves. It is about becoming curious rather than fearful, engaged rather than passive, and proactive rather than waiting for illness to dictate the next chapter of our lives.

No matter where you are starting from, the body remains remarkably responsive. The future is not determined solely by where you have been. It is influenced by what you choose next. I hope that these pages help you see your health differently, not as something that happens to you, but as something you help shape every single day.

Chapter 1

The Life We Learned to Call Normal

★★★

It is no measure of health to be well-adjusted to a profoundly sick society.
— Jiddu Krishnamurti

Something Felt Off

For a while, I believed health was mostly about doing the "right things." Eating reasonably well, exercising, going to medical appointments, following recommendations, trying harder, and remaining disciplined — all of it seemed like straightforward pieces of a formula that should eventually lead people toward wellness. I truly thought that if people followed the advice they were given, most of them would become healthier.

That is the framework many of us inherited. Health was presented as something relatively simple and linear. If someone was not well, the assumption frequently became that they were failing somewhere along the way — perhaps they lacked consistency, motivation, or self-control.

But over the years, something began unsettling me. Despite living in an extraordinarily medically advanced period in history, so many people still did not feel well. Not always catastrophically ill or carrying dramatic diagnoses, but quietly unwell in ways that seemed to permeate everyday life. People were running on empty, emotionally depleted, dependent on caffeine to function, unable to sleep deeply, constantly overwhelmed, and often carrying a strange underlying heaviness that had become so common it barely seemed noticeable anymore.

What affected me most was how individuals believed their suffering was a personal failure. The more patients I cared for, the more I began sensing something deeper beneath the symptoms. Many of these people were not lazy, weak, or lacking willpower. They were trying to survive in conditions their biology was struggling to keep up with.

And yet most people move through life without ever being taught how intricately everything inside us is connected. Instead, many of us learn to override the body rather than understand it. We suppress fatigue, push through stress, sleep less, consume more stimulation, ignore symptoms, and continue functioning until the body speaks louder. It can speak through burnout or anxiety, through inflammation, weight gain, chronic disease, or through the quiet feeling that something no longer feels right inside. I know that deep down, many of us can feel this, even if we cannot fully explain it. Some of us sense that modern life has drifted far beyond the conditions we evolved to navigate.

Part of my own awakening around health began the moment I stopped seeing symptoms as isolated problems and started asking a very different question: What if the body has been responding intelligently all along? Instead of viewing the body as something constantly malfunctioning, I began seeing it as something continuously adapting — trying to survive, compensate, and protect us, even when those adaptations become symptoms themselves.

And once I began seeing health through that lens, I could no longer look at medicine or the culture surrounding us in quite the same way again. Something fundamental had shifted not only in how I practiced, but in how I understood human beings.

The Patients I Couldn't Forget

One of the things medicine gives you, if you are paying attention, is a front-row seat to suffering. Not only physical suffering but suffering in all its complexity. You witness fear, shame, loneliness, frustration, and the quiet emotional burden people carry behind carefully composed appearances. Certain conversations began staying with me long after clinic hours ended.

I remember women sitting nervously on the exam table telling me, "I don't know what's wrong with me anymore. I don't feel like myself." I remember patients fighting tears because, despite eating less and trying harder, the scale continued climbing. Others laughed as they described how dependent they had become on caffeine to make it through the day.

What stood out most was how often people apologized for their weight and symptoms before I had even said a single word. As though struggling with their health had somehow become a moral failure.

Part of my work has also been as a nurse-midwife, caring for women during pregnancy and birth, years of life that should theoretically represent some of the healthiest and most resilient periods of the lifespan. However, what increasingly surprised me over the years working on the labor and delivery floor was how common metabolic dysfunction had become, even among women of childbearing age[1]. Gestational diabetes, hypertension, obesity, thyroid dysfunction, and complicated pregnancies were no longer unusual occurrences. What once stood out as acutely concerning slowly became expected simply because we were seeing it everywhere, all the time.

I also noticed how people felt profoundly alone in what they were experiencing, even as their symptoms had become ordinarily common. So many individuals believed they were somehow uniquely broken, while others around them were experiencing the same weariness, disconnection, frustration, and confusion.

Most importantly, I began to notice how desperately people were searching for understanding. They wanted someone to explain why they no longer felt like themselves. They wanted to understand why their energy had changed, why their metabolism felt different, why their sleep no longer felt restorative, or why they constantly felt as though they were fighting their own body.

The more I listened, the more I realized that many symptoms were not random failures of the body. They were opportunities. Messages carrying information about how someone had been living and what their physiology had been trying to manage for years. The body was not betraying them. It was just communicating.

And once I truly understood that, I could no longer approach health solely through the narrow lens of isolated symptoms and prescriptions. I became far more interested in patterns, physiology, root causes, and the environments shaping biology every single day. Without fully realizing it at first, I was waking up to a much bigger conversation.

A Different Way of Seeing

There was not one single moment that changed everything for me. The shift happened incrementally after thousands of patients, conversations, and observations.

The deeper I went into healthcare, the more I realized that most people had never been taught even the most basic principles about how the body actually works. No one had explained the extent to which daily life influences physiology, or how powerfully the body responds to repeated inputs over time. So many people were trying to function inside bodies they had never truly been taught to understand.

Once I realized that, my perspective as a clinician began changing. I became less interested in silencing symptoms and far more interested in helping people reconnect with the essential conditions their bodies had been asking for all along. This shift changed not only how I practiced, but how I lived. I began paying attention differently to my own energy, my own nervous system, and my own relationship with stress, rhythm, nourishment, rest, and presence. I came to understand something deeply humbling. Clinicians are not separate from the world we are trying to help people navigate. We are living inside it too.

This new perspective created even more compassion in me because healing stopped feeling like a conversation about perfection. It became a conversation about awareness. About learning how to listen earlier. About understanding that symptoms often carry information, and that even small shifts repeated consistently can reshape the trajectory of a life. That insight became one of the foundations of everything that followed.

Chapter 2

The Environment We Forget to Question

★★★

When a flower doesn't bloom, you fix the environment in which it grows, not the flower.
—Alexander Den Heijer

When Exhaustion Became Normal

There was a time when being tired used to mean something. It meant the body had worked hard, exerted itself, and now required recovery. Fatigue was once understood as a temporary state, a signal that rest was needed before balance could return. But somewhere along the way, exhaustion stopped being a message and became a lifestyle.

What unsettled me most was not how tired people had become, but how ordinary the tiredness now seemed. Everywhere I went, I heard some variation of the same conversation. People joked about surviving on caffeine, showed pride about sleeping only a few hours a night, and casually described levels of stress their bodies were clearly struggling to sustain. Fatigue had become so universally common that it no longer registered as a warning sign. It had become part of the culture.

I remember overhearing two women once while standing in line. One of them mentioned how unwell she had been for months, describing a kind of tiredness that went far beyond a busy week. Her friend smiled sympathetically and replied, "Well… welcome to the club." Both women laughed.

That moment stayed with me for a long time because of how ordinary it felt. There was no alarm in either of their voices. No sense that something might be wrong. Living in survival mode had become so widely accepted that people bonded over it casually, almost affectionately, as though feeling depleted was simply the unavoidable cost of adulthood.

That is one of the tragedies of our time: We have become so accustomed to surviving that we no longer remember what genuine vitality feels like.

The Water We Swim In

A concept that strongly influenced my thinking as a clinician is that human beings do not make choices in isolation. We are continuously shaped by the environments surrounding us — by what is available, marketed, rewarded, celebrated, and repeated every single day. Our habits are not formed in a vacuum. Neither are our food impulses, energy levels, emotional coping mechanisms, nor our relationship with food.

Sadly, far too many people blame themselves for struggles that make far more sense once the environment itself is examined more carefully. The world surrounding us constantly shapes behavior, often and invisibly. It influences how we eat, how we sleep, how we move, how we cope with stress, and even what we believe is "normal." These repeated exposures become so familiar that most individuals stop noticing them entirely. Like fish no longer notice the water they swim in.

The body absorbs life continuously, and once you truly start paying attention, it becomes impossible to ignore how profoundly today's environments pull us away from the conditions under which the body is most likely to thrive.

Food is available everywhere now. Not simply nourishment, but stimulation disguised as food. Gas stations, airports, waiting rooms, schools, office meetings, hospital cafeterias, checkout counters, sporting events, pharmacies, vending machines — nearly every space people move through is saturated with ultra-processed convenience foods specifically designed to be hyper-palatable, rapidly rewarding, inexpensive, and difficult to stop eating[2]. And because this surrounds us constantly, we no longer detect how unusual it truly is.

Children now grow up surrounded by brightly colored marketing, sugary drinks, processed snacks,[3] oversized portions, and foods engineered to capture attention long before they are old enough to understand what is happening at a biological level.

The nutritional landscape has changed dramatically in a relatively short time. Our biology did not evolve for continuous exposure to hyper-processed foods[4], constant notifications, artificial light, sedentary living, chronic stress, and uninterrupted stimulation. The body still operates largely on ancient biological systems shaped around movement, natural rhythms, sunlight, periods of scarcity, real food, sleep, and recovery. Today's life often provides the opposite. And the mismatch is profound.

A Nervous System That Never Rests

Once I began noticing this pattern, I saw it everywhere. People moved through their days overstimulated, overfed yet undernourished, wired and worn down yet unable to truly rest. Even moments that appear restful are saturated with mental input. A person might sit on the couch at the end of a long day, but their nervous system is still flooded with notifications, television, scrolling, background noise, and the subtle pressure to remain engaged at all times. Life rarely allows the nervous system to fully exhale, since we are always mentally rehearsing the next obligation.

The nervous system was never designed for constant input, yet a growing number of people now live inside uninterrupted streams of information, urgency, comparison, and low-grade stress. Our physiology carries the imprint of all of it.

The body adapts to this environment remarkably well. Stress hormones such as adrenaline, noradrenaline, and cortisol rise[5]. Sleep becomes lighter and less restorative. Attention fragments while food urges intensify, and anxiety slowly becomes baseline.

And because these changes happen gradually, the connection between how we live and how we feel often goes unnoticed. People assume the fatigue means they are lazy. The cravings mean they lack discipline. The anxiety feels personal. The weight gain feels inexplicable. Brain fog becomes something they try to push through. So, I began to wonder whether many of these struggles made far more sense when viewed through the lens of the environments people lived in every day.

The Handrails We Lost

I think about this often when I reflect on the differences between my upbringing in Spain and the food environment I later encountered in the United States. My childhood was certainly not nutritionally perfect. Processed foods and sugary pastries existed. Convenience foods were becoming increasingly common. I became keenly attached to carbohydrates and blood sugar instability long before I fully understood metabolism.

But despite all of that, there were still handrails. Homemade meals eaten sitting down together at the table were the norm. Vegetables and non-processed protein were part of daily life. Fast food existed, but it had not yet fully become woven into the rhythm of everyday eating. Drinking multiple sodas every day would have felt excessive. Constant snacking throughout the day would not have seemed ordinary. I did not fully appreciate those handrails until much later.

When I moved to the United States, I remember feeling almost overwhelmed by the sheer intensity of the food environment. Portion sizes were larger[6]. Sugary drinks were everywhere. Convenience dominated daily life. Meals could consist almost entirely of ultra-processed carbohydrates, refined oils, packaged snacks, and highly engineered foods designed for repeated consumption.

At the same time, life itself seemed faster. People ate while driving, multitasking, standing, working, rushing between obligations, or staring at screens. Snacking became constant. Convenience replaced rhythm. And because entire generations grew up inside this environment, much of it stopped feeling unusual.

That normalization is one of the most important ideas in this book because we are trying to create healthy bodies inside environments that inadvertently promote metabolic chaos. A great deal of suffering stems not from lack of discipline, but from environments that push biology in difficult directions.

The Great Nutritional Confusion

One of the saddest realities of today's eating trends is that well-intentioned individuals genuinely believe they are making good choices as they try to navigate an increasingly complex nutritional landscape.

Most people do not intentionally harm themselves or their families. They trust the systems, recommendations, advertisements, and food culture surrounding them. Parents pass down the knowledge they have. Families repeat the patterns they inherited. Entire societies have adopted ways of eating that the body often struggles to tolerate for long periods. That understanding removed a great deal of judgment from the way I view health.

For decades, nutritional messaging has become increasingly contradictory. Fat became feared. "Low-fat" products flooded grocery stores. Sugar quietly replaced fat in a myriad of foods while still being marketed as healthy. Convenience products were presented under the guise of wellness, and people gradually became disconnected from the simplicity of real nourishment while increasingly overloading their bodies with unhealthy food.

At the same time, nutrition has become increasingly reduced to labels, marketing claims, percentages, calorie counting, and constantly changing headlines. While one expert promotes a low-fat diet, another promotes high-carbohydrate eating, meal replacements, detoxes, supplements, or extreme restrictions. Social media amplifies the noise even further, creating an endless stream of conflicting advice that leaves people feeling more overwhelmed than informed.

Among all these contradictory messages, many people stop trusting themselves completely. They no longer know what to believe, whom to trust, or how to make sense of food in a way that feels sustainable.

That is one reason simplicity matters so much. Because, despite all the noise surrounding nutrition, the body still responds remarkably well to real nourishment.

The Signals We Learn to Ignore

What concerns me most is how disconnected people have become from their own internal signals. Many ignore hunger until they are ravenous, ignore fatigue until they crash, ignore stress until anxiety surfaces physically, and ignore emotional strain until numbness replaces feeling altogether.

The body whispers first, then nudges, then interrupts, and eventually forces attention. But the culture surrounding us trains people to override nearly every stage of that communication. Push through. Keep going. Drink more coffee. Stay productive. Don't fall behind.

I wondered what would happen if people became quiet long enough to truly listen to what their body had been trying to say for years.

Because beneath many symptoms, there is usually a deeper story about how someone has been living, not only physically, but emotionally too. The body is not irrational, but it gets forced to adapt. The overextended body slows down because it needs restoration. The anxious mind becomes hypervigilant when the nervous system no longer feels consistently safe. The insulin-resistant system attempts to manage constant metabolic overload[7]. The inflamed cells respond to repeated physiological strain. All of this is the body's attempt to communicate, but the problem is that we have spent years being taught not to listen.

I often think of symptoms the way I think about warning lights on a car dashboard. When a fuel light turns on, the car owner does not become angry at the light. They understand that the light provides useful information about something that requires attention. The light itself is not the problem. It is the messenger. Our bodies work much the same way. Far too often, symptoms are treated as though they are the problem. But in reality, they are more like dashboard warning lights, drawing our attention toward something deeper that may need to be uncovered.

Chapter 3

We Learned to Wait for Disease

★★★

The doctor of the future will give no medicine but will interest patients in the care of the human frame, in diet, and in the cause and prevention of disease.
— Thomas Edison

The Waiting Room

There is something strangely symbolic about a medical waiting room. People sit quietly beneath fluorescent lights, holding clipboards, medication lists, insurance cards, and fears they often have not fully spoken aloud yet. Some are waiting for reassurance. Others are waiting for answers. Many are waiting to discover whether something serious is happening inside their body while hoping the news will somehow restore a sense of safety and certainty again.

In many ways, that waiting room reflects the philosophy healthcare inherited for generations. Symptoms appear, diseases progress unnoticed for years, and eventually the body becomes loud enough that intervention can no longer be postponed. Medicine then steps in to diagnose, stabilize, repair, treat, or manage what has already fully emerged.

To be fair, medicine has become extraordinarily skilled at intervention. We now survive infections, injuries, surgeries, and illnesses that would have been devastating only a century ago. Advances in technology, pharmaceuticals, emergency medicine, imaging, and surgical care have transformed countless lives and saved millions of people. I deeply respect medicine, and I participate in it every day. But alongside those extraordinary achievements, another reality emerges.

Traditional medicine is often far less skilled at recognizing the slow erosion of vitality before dysfunction becomes severe enough to fit neatly into a diagnosis. Most chronic illnesses do not appear suddenly. The body rarely moves overnight from vibrant health into severe disease. Much of what eventually becomes visible develops gradually through years of accumulated physiological change, long before catastrophe finally announces itself. Blood sugar regulation may begin to deteriorate, sleep becomes less restorative, and muscle mass slowly declines. Inflammation rises quietly in the background while energy becomes less reliable and recovery takes longer than it once did. Waistlines expand so gradually that the change often goes unnoticed. Because these shifts occur little by little, they rarely create a sense of urgency. Then one day, a diagnosis appears, and it suddenly feels as though disease arrived out of nowhere.

The Fifteen-Minute Appointment

There is something painful about caring for human beings inside a system that leaves so little time for actual conversations. Most healthcare providers enter medicine because they genuinely want to help people heal. They study for years, sacrifice enormously, and carry tremendous responsibility. Yet once inside the system, many quickly discover that healthcare often functions under relentless pressure. Visits become shorter, documentation grows endlessly, insurance restrictions shape decisions, and administrative demands consume increasing amounts of time and emotional energy.

Meanwhile, patients arrive carrying lives far more complicated than any brief appointment could possibly hold. A woman may come into her clinic appointment exhausted, stressed, with brain fog, unstable blood sugar, and emotionally overloaded. Yet by the time medications are reviewed, forms are completed, and labs are discussed, the clock runs out, with no time left to begin exploring what her body has truly been navigating for years.

The system naturally gravitates toward symptom management because symptoms are measurable, immediate, and easier to address quickly. Preserving health requires something much slower and far more relational: context, pattern recognition, education, prevention, meaningful conversations, and trust. Above all, it takes time, which is one of the things modern healthcare often has the least of.

What We Are Taught

One of the things that became increasingly clear to me over the years is that most healthcare providers were trained primarily to recognize, diagnose, and treat disease. That is not a criticism of medicine. It is simply the structure in which many of us were educated.

In school, enormous amounts of time are dedicated to pathology, pharmacology, diagnosis, treatment protocols, complications, and learning which medications correspond to which conditions. We learn how to intervene once the disease is present. But curricula dedicate relatively little time teaching how to preserve health long before dysfunction appears.

There is surprisingly little discussion about metabolic health, muscle preservation, sleep quality, nervous system regulation, ultra-processed foods, insulin resistance, chronic inflammation, or the cumulative physiological impact of contemporary living patterns over decades. Nutrition education itself[8] is often minimal despite the enormous role food plays in long-term health outcomes[9].

And because healthcare providers care deeply about their patients, most continue practicing within the framework they were taught. Patients arrive with symptoms, diagnoses are made, medications are prescribed, and the current disease is managed as effectively as possible.

The problem is that by the time many chronic conditions become obvious enough to be diagnosed clearly, dysfunction has been developing silently for years. This made me question why healthcare tends to wait for the disease to become advanced before mobilizing aggressively, instead of placing far greater attention on preserving health earlier, while the body is still highly adaptable and resilient.

The Pharmaceutical Influence

As I moved deeper into clinical practice, I also began noticing how strongly the healthcare system gravitates toward pharmaceutical solutions. Medications save lives. Many are incredibly valuable and, for some conditions, absolutely essential. Unfortunately, they usually enter the picture long before lifestyle factors are fully explored.

A patient develops elevated blood pressure, and medication becomes part of the discussion. As time passes, blood sugar or cholesterol levels rise, sleep quality declines, anxiety becomes more prominent, or bone loss begins to emerge. Each new concern is often met with an additional treatment aimed at the currently visible problem. While these interventions may be appropriate and sometimes necessary, the underlying physiological changes that may have been unfolding quietly for years often receive far less attention than the symptoms they eventually produce.

Also, many patients receive medications for conditions whose roots extend far beyond a single organ because healthcare frequently separates symptoms into isolated compartments. The result is that patients often spend years managing disease without ever fully understanding what may have contributed to it in the first place.

Learning to Preserve Health

A significant shift in my thinking came when I understood that preserving health is not the same thing as detecting disease early. For many years, healthcare has increasingly incorporated preventive screening into routine care. Physical exams, mammograms, colonoscopies, Pap smears, blood pressure monitoring, cholesterol testing, and other screenings have unquestionably saved many lives by helping detect disease earlier.

But I came to observe that much of what we call preventive care is still designed to identify dysfunction after physiological changes have been unfolding beneath the surface for years or even decades.

A colonoscopy may detect colon cancer earlier, but it does not necessarily address why that person developed polyps or disease in the first place. Our healthcare still functions downstream, intervening once dysfunction is already developing rather than placing greater emphasis on upstream prevention and preserving health long before disease emerges[10]. That distinction changed the way I thought about health entirely. I became increasingly interested in helping people preserve optimal function. How do we help people maintain metabolic health, strength, energy, mobility, resilience, cognitive function, and emotional well-being over decades rather than waiting for decline to force attention?

That question reshaped how I viewed medicine, prevention, aging, and the relationship between humans and their bodies. Because true prevention is not simply about finding disease sooner. It is about creating the conditions that make disease less likely to develop.

Chapter 4

Nourishment Made Simple

★★★

If it came from a plant, eat it.
If it was made in a plant, don't.
— Michael Pollan

The Noise Around Food

By this point, we have explored how significantly our environment shapes how we eat, crave, choose, and cope. Nutrition has become increasingly complicated with endless debates about the "right" way to eat. The result is not clarity but overwhelm. Eating no longer feels intuitive. Meals become something to analyze, second-guess, restrict, or control rather than a simple act of nourishment. Somewhere along the way, people have lost touch with what it feels like to eat in a way that truly supports their health. Despite the complexity of nutrition, relatively simple changes can have a profound impact.

Personally, and clinically, I have watched people improve not because they followed extreme dietary philosophies, but because they simplified their eating enough for their bodies to finally function with less noise.

What Are We Calling Food?

Most people would not spend a fortune on a high-end vehicle and then deliberately fill it with the wrong fuel. We understand intuitively that performance depends on what powers the machine. If someone purchased a luxury sports car, they would carefully follow the manufacturer's recommendations to keep the vehicle running at its best. Yet many of us approach our bodies very differently.

The body is infinitely more sophisticated than any machine we will ever own. However, we often expect it to function optimally regardless of the quality of the fuel we provide. We are surprised by how we feel while rarely questioning whether we are supplying the raw materials it needs to perform well. Food is more than calories. It is information. And just as fuel influences how a high-performance engine runs, nutrition influences how every cell functions.

One of the simplest ways I have learned to think about nourishment is this: We are designed to recognize real food. That does not mean every person must eat the same way, nor does it mean nutrition needs to become rigid or obsessive. We thrive on different foods, cultures, traditions, preferences, and lifestyles. Despite disagreements over nutrition, certain patterns emerge in healthier dietary approaches worldwide. Meals centered on protein, vegetables, fiber, healthy fats, minimally processed carbohydrates, and foods that still resemble their original form tend to provide far greater stability than diets dominated by industrialized products.

Many modern food products have become so normalized that people have stopped questioning what they actually are. For years, margarine was marketed as a healthier alternative to butter. People genuinely believed they were making a healthier choice by replacing a traditional food with a highly industrialized product largely made from processed vegetable oils chemically altered to remain solid at room temperature. Some of these products contained partially hydrogenated oils, now strongly associated with inflammation, cardiovascular disease, and metabolic dysfunction[11].

For decades, families were taught to view heavily processed breakfast cereals as healthy daily nutrition for children. Brightly colored options loaded with refined sugars, artificial flavors, additives, and rapidly absorbed carbohydrates were aggressively marketed as part of a "balanced breakfast," often paired with fat-free milk at a time when low-fat eating was heavily promoted. People trusted marketing more than their own intuition.

In *Metabolical*, physician and researcher Robert Lustig argues that many industrialized food products are designed less around nourishment and more around shelf life, hyper-palatability, and maximizing consumption. Food is no longer organized around physiology, but around industrial efficiency and profitability[12].

The Carbohydrates and Fat Debate

An unfortunate development in contemporary nutrition is that conversations about food have become increasingly reductionist. Nutrients have been isolated, simplified, and turned into ideological battles rather than understood through the lens of metabolic health. First, fat became feared, and then carbohydrates became demonized. Entire groups of foods were labeled as universally "good" or "bad," while nuance disappeared from the conversation.

A common example of this is the misunderstanding surrounding low-carbohydrate nutrition. When experts recommend reducing carbohydrates, they are generally not referring to fiber-rich vegetables such as leafy greens, broccoli, cauliflower, asparagus, zucchini, and other minimally processed plant foods. These foods tend to have a relatively modest impact on blood sugar and provide important nutrients and fiber. More commonly, the recommendation focuses on limiting carbohydrates that rapidly raise blood glucose, including refined sugars, sweetened beverages, pastries, breads, processed cereals, refined grains, and other highly processed starches.

And even here, context still matters enormously. Some carbohydrates that are generally considered nutritious, such as whole-grain rice, oats, quinoa, potatoes, and beans, may still behave very differently depending on an individual's metabolic health.

An insulin-sensitive and physically active person often tolerates these foods very differently than someone experiencing insulin resistance, prediabetes, obesity, or longstanding metabolic dysfunction[13]. Such an individual may temporarily require a significantly lower carbohydrate intake in order to stabilize blood sugar, reduce insulin demand, and help restore metabolic health.

This is one of the reasons nutrition conversations have become so difficult to navigate. People began searching for universal dietary rules in situations where individual needs vary tremendously.

A similar narrative emerged with dietary fat. For years, fat itself was portrayed as something inherently dangerous. Grocery stores became filled with low-fat products marketed as healthier alternatives, many of which compensated for the loss of fat by dramatically increasing sugars, refined starches, additives, artificial flavors, and other highly processed ingredients to preserve taste and texture.

During the height of the low-fat era, consumers were encouraged to avoid foods such as eggs, butter, full-fat yogurt, and naturally occurring fats in meat. At the same time, they were consuming an increasing number of processed fat-free products that often provided far less satiety and metabolic stability.

Part of the problem was that discussions about fat rarely distinguished between different types of fats. Naturally occurring fats found in whole and minimally processed foods became grouped together with highly processed industrial oils, despite their very different effects on health. Yet the body does not respond to all fats in the same way. It responds very differently to oils that have been heavily refined and repeatedly exposed to high heat than it does to fats that occur naturally in food. Healthy fats play essential roles in hormone production, brain function, cell membrane integrity, nutrient absorption, and helping meals feel satisfying and metabolically stable.

One example I frequently discuss with patients is yogurt. Many people believe they are making a healthier choice by purchasing fat-free flavored yogurts. Yet once fat is removed, these products often contain large amounts of added sugar without the balancing effects that fat normally provides. The result is a product marketed as "healthy" that may still contribute to significant blood sugar instability.

Nutrition becomes far simpler when we stop viewing foods through the lens of rigid dietary ideology and begin looking at how they function in the body. Real food consistently provides signals that support health, while heavily processed products often create the opposite effect.

Protein Creates Stability

If there is one nutritional shift that consistently changes how people feel, it is appropriately increasing protein intake. Today's dietary norms have become remarkably protein-poor, with little awareness of this trend. Breakfast often consists of coffee and refined carbohydrates. Lunch turns into whatever is fast and convenient. Dinner frequently arrives after long, draining days, when blood sugar is already unstable and has already affected decision-making. People are technically consuming more than enough calories while chronically under-consuming one of the body's most important nutritional building blocks.

One of the conversations I have repeatedly in clinic is helping people rethink what constitutes a nourishing meal. Many individuals have spent years calling something food that, metabolically, was primarily a large amount of refined carbohydrates with very little else to support metabolic stability. Donuts with sugary coffee for breakfast. A sandwich and chips for lunch, and pizza for dinner are simply not nutritionally balanced choices. There is a profound difference between a plate built primarily around rapidly absorbed carbohydrates and one built around protein, vegetables, and healthy fats.

A simple visual framework I often teach patients is to build a protein-forward plate. Ideally, a generous portion of the plate comes from fiber-rich vegetables, a substantial portion is centered on protein, and carbohydrates play a smaller, intentional role rather than taking over the entire meal.

Protein matters because it helps create lasting satiety. It slows the return of hunger. It supports steadier energy. It helps the body feel more satisfied, rather than constantly searching for the next snack.

This becomes especially important for women, who are traditionally taught to eat lightly, restrict calories, and choose foods that appear "healthy" but leave them physiologically undernourished. Many women spend years eating breakfasts without enough substance, salads without enough protein, or small meals that look virtuous but do not actually support stable energy, hormones, strength, or appetite regulation.

Consistently, patients notice how little protein they had been consuming for years. Interestingly, the traditional recommended dietary allowance (RDA) for protein remains approximately 0.8 grams per kilogram of body weight per day, a number originally designed primarily to prevent deficiency rather than optimize metabolic health[14].

In recent years, an increasing number of clinicians have argued that many adults are likely to benefit from significantly higher protein intake. Conservative research shows that an intake of approximately 1.2–1.6 grams per kilogram of body weight may better support metabolic health, appetite regulation, recovery, and the preservation of lean body mass over time[14].

A Simple Experiment

After years of watching people struggle despite their best efforts, one lesson kept emerging: My patients no longer needed more nutritional theory. They needed clarity.

This became one of the inspirations behind creating my online 5-Day Gut Reset Program (see end of Chapter 10). The program's intention was for participants to reduce interference enough to make the underlying signals easier to appreciate. What struck me most was not only how quickly participants noticed physical changes, but how emotional some of those discoveries became.

Several participants described feeling calmer around food for the first time in years. Others noticed that cravings softened dramatically after only a few days of reducing processed foods and stabilizing meals around more recognizable nourishment. Many began to see how much of their eating had been driven by depletion, convenience, emotional habits, or unstable blood sugar rather than true hunger itself.

One participant shared that she went camping during the Reset and fully expected the trip to derail her progress. Instead, she found that she could still nourish herself differently while enjoying the weekend, and for the first time, she no longer felt controlled by the snacks surrounding her.

Another participant shared her experience overflowing with excitement. She and her husband had spent the weekend traveling and attending a concert, exactly the kind of situation where healthy choices become almost impossible. And yet she explained that her relationship with food had shifted. Instead of automatically overeating or choosing food mindlessly out of habit, they found themselves making wiser decisions. They also shared meals at restaurants and still felt completely satisfied. One unexpected thing she mentioned, almost jokingly, was that restaurant meals had become significantly less expensive because they were no longer ordering far more food than they could eat.

What stayed with me most about these conversations was the sense of relief people described. Nourishment had stopped feeling like a battle. Many participants realized that eating differently did not require obsession, punishment, or endless willpower. Once the body became more stable, hunger often felt calmer, cravings became quieter, and meals became more satisfying than before. It was eye-opening to witness how powerfully the body responds when we simply stop constantly overwhelming it.

Leading the 5-Day Gut Reset left a lasting impression on me. The questions it generated revealed that people were searching not only for better health but also for a clearer understanding of why their bodies were struggling in the first place. That realization became the foundation for everything that followed. It inspired the writing of this book and eventually evolved into the 28-Day Metabolic Restoration Program presented in Chapter 10— a practical roadmap designed to help readers move from understanding foundational nutrition principles to putting them into practice.

Chapter 5

The Truth About Sugar

★★★

Sugar is the new tobacco.
— Robert Lustig

The Sweetest Trap

Part of what makes sugar so deceptive is that it rarely enters people's lives looking dangerous. It arrives wrapped in comfort, celebration, convenience, reward, childhood memories, and emotional relief. It appears during birthdays, holidays, school events, road trips, office meetings, sports games, stressful afternoons, and late nights when fatigue lowers resistance and quick comfort feels irresistible.

Sugar becomes woven into life so thoroughly that it stops feeling like a substance at all and passes largely unquestioned. It is no longer an occasional indulgence. It has become a constant presence in the modern food environment.

Over a hundred years ago, the average person consumed only a small fraction of the sugar consumed today. Current estimates suggest that the average American consumes well over one hundred pounds of added sugar each year, an amount that would have been difficult for previous generations[15] to imagine.

The World Health Organization recommends ideally keeping added sugar intake below approximately twenty-five grams per day for meaningful health benefits[16]. Meanwhile, a single regular twelve-ounce soda often contains nearly forty grams of sugar on its own.

One drink, one ordinary moment, and already the body is being asked to process more sugar than many experts recommend for an entire day. Once people begin seeing those numbers clearly, it becomes easier to understand why blood sugar instability, insulin resistance, and metabolic dysfunction have become so widespread.

What makes this even more complicated is that sugar affects far more than weight. It influences energy, appetite, focus, emotional regulation, hunger, and sleep in ways that are grossly underestimated. And because those effects happen repeatedly over time, people fail to grasp the relationship between how they feel and what their physiology is being exposed to every single day. Meanwhile, their biology may be riding repeated waves of glucose spikes and crashes from morning until night.

The Crashes That Became My Identity

When I reflect on my own relationship with sugar growing up, I realize how unstable blood sugar swings had become part of who I was long before I understood the science behind it. For decades, I was convinced that I could not function without carbohydrates. I always needed snacks nearby. Leaving the house without food was unthinkable because I genuinely believed I might "crash" if too much time passed between meals. If I became hungry, I would feel shaky, irritable, anxious, emotionally overwhelmed, and unable to think clearly. I was convinced I had hypoglycemia.

My issues with hunger became so familiar that the people around me learned to recognize it too. We even developed a simple system. If I announced that I was hungry, they would ask, "What number are you?" We used a scale from zero to ten to describe how urgent the situation felt. A zero meant completely satisfied. A ten meant I needed food immediately. At the time, I never questioned any of it. That way of living felt normal; it had become part of my identity.

People often normalize the very symptoms their body has been trying to communicate for years. I did not understand that my energy was unstable or that my physiology was constantly swinging between glucose spikes and crashes. And I certainly did not understand how profoundly food was affecting how I felt emotionally and physically throughout the day.

Everything began to change after I upgraded my nutrition at almost 50 years old. To my surprise, the constant preoccupation with hunger disappeared. For the first time in my adult life, I could go longer periods without eating and remain calm, clear-headed, and functional. What I learned was that I had not conquered hunger. I had developed greater metabolic flexibility. I had become better at accessing stored energy rather than relying almost exclusively on a constant supply of sugar and carbohydrates. The freedom that came with that shift was striking.

Looking back, I am amazed at how common that experience may be, without people fully seeing that they may be trapped in repeated cycles of metabolic instability. And the difficult part is that once someone adapts to those cycles long enough, they stop recognizing how chaotic they actually feel internally.

The Body Reacts Honestly

A particularly memorable reminder of this happened unexpectedly one afternoon while I was out with my fifteen-year-old son after he had been practicing driving.

He wanted to stop at a tea shop he enjoys, and because I happened to be wearing a continuous glucose monitor at the time, I decided to turn the moment into a small personal experiment. Normally, I would not order one of those drinks for myself. But that day, I chose the same tea he ordered, except I specifically requested mine with fifty percent less sugar than the regular version. In my mind, I was convinced I was making a fairly reasonable choice. What happened afterward shocked me. My glucose spiked to nearly 300 mg/dL.

Watching the graph climb on my phone transformed an abstract concept into something immediate and visible. I already understood blood sugar intellectually. But seeing my own body respond in real time made the experience feel entirely different.

What affected me most was realizing how common those glucose surges are throughout the day, often occurring without people ever seeing them. Then, a few hours later, they feel shaky, foggy, irritable, hungry again, emotionally unstable, or desperate for another source of quick energy — without understanding that their body is responding exactly as it was designed to respond. Once you begin seeing those patterns clearly, it becomes difficult to unsee them[17].

Cravings Are Not Character Flaws

Among the most heartbreaking things I see clinically is the amount of shame people carry around food. I have sat with patients who lowered their voices when talking about sugar, almost as though confessing something deeply embarrassing. Some described feeling completely out of control around certain foods. Others talk about hiding snacks, eating in secret, or promising themselves every morning that "this time" they will finally have more discipline.

In many cases, compulsive sugar eating is not a character flaw at all, but the predictable consequence of repeatedly exposing the brain to highly stimulating foods engineered specifically to keep people wanting more. Researchers continue debating exactly how addictive sugar truly is compared to substances like nicotine or drugs, but there is little doubt that highly processed sugary foods strongly activate reward pathways in the brain[18]. And once people understand that, shame often begins loosening its grip. Not because responsibility disappears. But because clarity enters the conversation for the first time.

The Sugar-Free Illusion

I commonly hear patients say: "I do not really drink soda anymore... only diet soda." This common response reflects how we have come to view artificial sweeteners as a harmless substitute for sugar. Yet that assumption raises an important question: What happens when the brain and palate remain constantly exposed to intensely sweet flavors even in the absence of calories?

Research continues evolving in this area, but growing evidence suggests that certain artificial sweeteners may still influence cravings, appetite regulation, insulin responses, the gut microbiome, and the brain's relationship with sweetness itself[19]. In other words, even when calories disappear, the impact can still be highly detrimental. Many artificially sweetened products continue reinforcing the same attachment to hyper-sweet taste that helped create metabolic instability in the first place.

This is one of the reasons I strongly encourage patients to gradually retrain their palates rather than replacing sugar with endless artificial substitutes. The objective is not only to reduce sugar intake but also to reduce dependence on extreme sweetness itself.

When that advice is followed, something unexpected happens. Foods that once tasted perfectly balanced begin tasting overwhelmingly sweet[20]. Eventually, products that were once consumed daily — sodas, sweetened coffees, desserts, processed snacks — no longer even taste good to them because their perception of taste has fundamentally shifted. What once felt difficult begins to feel effortless.

Not all sweeteners behave the same. More natural alternatives, such as stevia, monk fruit, and allulose, may be better for some individuals, particularly when used in less-processed forms without additional additives or artificial ingredients. Personally, allulose has become one of my preferred options because it behaves much more like sugar while having far less impact on blood sugar.

Chapter 6

Muscle Changes Everything

★★★

Never forget: Strength preserves freedom.
—Vanessa Menanteau

The Gym Membership I Barely Used

For much of my life, my relationship with exercise has moved in cycles. There were periods when I felt energized and deeply connected to movement, and other periods when exercise felt distant, forced, or exhausting before I had even begun. About three years ago, I went through a phase where I was incredibly active. I played pickleball constantly, went hiking, rode bikes, and really enjoyed it all. Activity felt natural during that season of my life. It brought energy, lightness, and momentum into my days.

Then life shifted, the way it often does. My focus moved toward other responsibilities, other interests, other emotional needs, and movement began slipping further into the background again. I still understood how important exercise was. By that point, I was already completely immersed in the longevity world and fully aware of the enormous role muscle plays in metabolic health, aging, insulin sensitivity, cognitive preservation, and long-term vitality[21]. I knew the science very well. But knowledge alone does not always create action.

I had a membership to a beautiful gym. For a while, I would go consistently, convincing myself that this time things would finally stick.

Then, little by little, I would stop going, even while the monthly membership continued to be charged to my account. Years would pass before I finally canceled, carrying with me the strange guilt that comes from knowing something matters deeply while still struggling to integrate it fully into my own life. That disconnect humbled me. Because it made me realize how common that tension has become. Individuals understand movement matters. They want to feel stronger, healthier, more energized, and more capable in their own bodies. But wanting something intellectually and finding a sustainable rhythm emotionally are two very different things. For a long time, I believed motivation was the missing piece. Later, I realized the real issue was much more nuanced than that.

The Body Wants to Conserve Energy

One of the things medicine teaches you over time is that we are extraordinarily adaptive. A body that feels depleted, overwhelmed, inflamed, under-recovered, emotionally burdened, sleep-deprived, or metabolically unstable does not naturally crave exertion. It often craves conservation. It is easy to interpret resistance as laziness or a lack of discipline when the body may be trying to conserve energy in the best way it can while keeping up with the demands of work, responsibility, stress, and the emotional weight that builds throughout adulthood.

Some people remain there for years. They wake up exhausted, move through their day overstimulated and mentally overloaded, then blame themselves for not having the desire to perform at the gym afterward. The body begins to associate exercise with one more demand rather than something restorative or life-giving.

And yet movement is not punishment for having a body. Movement is one of the ways the body remembers itself. Therefore, it is important to start paying closer attention to which kinds of movement actually leave you feeling alive afterward rather than depleted. That distinction makes a significant difference.

The Unexpected Turning Point

For me, the shift happened in a way I did not anticipate. As I was preparing the material for our virtual 5-day Gut Reset Program, I decided that I wanted participants to have simple movement options available each day alongside the nutritional guidance. Before recommending any of the home exercise videos, I tested them myself to ensure they felt approachable, effective, and realistic for beginners.

Something unexpected happened during that process. I started enjoying exercise again. I found myself looking forward to certain workouts and noticing how different I felt afterward, not only physically, but emotionally and mentally too.

For me, the breakthrough came from discovering forms of movement that felt engaging rather than obligatory. For the first time in years, Tabata, Pilates, HIIT workouts, yoga, and home-based strength felt accessible in a way traditional gyms never consistently had. I realized that one of my biggest barriers for years was not movement itself. It was the process of leaving the house, driving somewhere, navigating the gym, and forcing exercise into a structure that no longer fit my life's rhythm.

The key to long-term success is that exercise becomes dramatically easier to sustain once it feels compatible with life instead of constantly fighting against it. Once that obstacle disappeared for me, consistency became far more achievable.

At the same time, I began understanding something important that applies far beyond my own experience: Movement does not need to look a certain way to make a considerable impact. Far too many individuals spend years believing exercise only "counts" if it happens inside a gym, follows a perfect routine, or resembles the intense fitness culture constantly presented on social media. That belief alone discourages would-be exercisers before they even begin.

One of the biggest misconceptions about exercise is that meaningful results require countless hours in the gym. Fortunately, research paints a much more encouraging picture. For most people, especially those just getting started, two resistance-training sessions per week can provide most of the strength, muscle, mobility, and metabolic benefits they seek.

In other words, you do not need to exercise perfectly to benefit tremendously. In most cases, it is not about optimization, but participation and consistency[22].

For some people, the first sustainable step may be walking outside every morning. For others, it may be Pilates in the living room, a short at-home strength workout, dancing, yoga, hiking, cycling, or simply moving more throughout the day. The most important thing is not finding the perfect exercise plan. It is finding forms of movement that feel realistic enough to repeat consistently. The specific form matters less than the relationship being built with movement itself.

Once you begin experiencing the benefits firsthand, something starts shifting naturally. Energy, strength, mood, and even sleep often improve. You begin feeling more capable, more stable, and more alive. Eventually, movement stops feeling like punishment and starts feeling supportive. It stops feeling like one more demand imposed from the outside and starts becoming something the body genuinely wants more of. That is where change truly begins.

Strength Is Protection

For many years, exercise was presented to people almost entirely through the lens of appearance. The conversation centered around becoming thinner, burning calories, fitting into smaller clothes, or changing how the body looked externally. Very little attention was given to what strength protects internally. But muscle changes far more than appearance.

Muscle influences metabolic health, blood sugar regulation, stability, balance, bone strength, mobility, recovery, and resilience during illness or injury[23]. It becomes increasingly important with age because strength determines not only how long someone lives but also how well they live as they age[24].

That reality became deeply personal for me at the end of 2025 when my father, who was eighty years old at the time, slipped near the pool at the gym and fractured his femur. An injury like that at that age can completely change the trajectory of a person's life. Recovery after major fractures becomes far more difficult as people grow older, especially when muscle mass, mobility, and physical resilience are already declining. Hip fractures in older adults are associated with remarkably high mortality rates within the following year, partly because not everyone fully regains their strength, independence, or mobility afterward[25].

When I received the call about my father's accident, of course, I was worried. But very quickly another thought entered my mind: If anyone was physically prepared to face something this difficult, it was him. My father exercised consistently for most of his life. He lifted weights, swam regularly, stayed active, and treated movement as part of his typical rhythm for decades. Even at eighty, he was still running his architecture firm while spending hours at the gym each day. And that strength mattered enormously once the injury happened.

After the required surgery, he had the upper-body strength to move himself, support himself with crutches, and regain mobility much faster than most adults his age could have. His recovery was still difficult, painful, and emotionally challenging, but his body had reserves to draw from. He had spent years building resilience long before he ever needed it.

That experience reinforced something longevity medicine teaches over and over again: Strength becomes incredibly important when life suddenly becomes hard. People rarely build muscle thinking about future injuries, surgeries, illnesses, or recovery. But the body remembers the investment. Muscle becomes a kind of physiological savings account that people draw from during periods of stress, aging, hospitalization, or physical adversity.

The most hopeful part is that the body remains adaptable for far longer than we assume. Strength can improve at almost any age[26]. The same goes for balance, mobility, and energy. The body continues responding to repeated signals of movement and resistance even later in life.

Muscle has been described as the body's longevity organ par excellence. It supports metabolic health, preserves independence, strengthens resilience, and helps carry us through the inevitable challenges of aging. Strength is not something we build for today. It is something we invest in for the future version of ourselves. And one day, often when we least expect it, we may be grateful that we started building it long before we needed it.

Chapter 7

Labs Don't Lie

★★★

Facts do not cease to exist because they are ignored.
— Aldous Huxley

Why "Normal" Is Not Always Optimal

The body rarely moves abruptly from health to illness. Chronic diseases develop gradually through patterns that accumulate over years. Understanding this progression transforms lab results from isolated numbers into windows that can offer a glimpse of what is happening beneath the surface. They become another way to pick up subtle changes long before symptoms become impossible to ignore. The body whispers long before it screams. And when interpreted thoughtfully and placed into the larger context of a person's life, laboratory trends can reveal those whispers surprisingly early.

One of the things I hear most often is patients being told, "Your labs look normal." At times, those words bring reassurance. Other times, they leave people feeling even more confused than before. I have sat across from patients describing endless symptoms and the persistent feeling that something inside them no longer feels right. Many had already seen multiple providers before arriving in my office. Most had been told some variation of the same thing: everything appears fine. And yet they did not feel fine.

A typically misunderstood aspect of laboratory testing is the meaning of the word "normal." Most people understandably assume that if laboratory results fall within the reference range, everything must be functioning properly. But laboratory ranges are based on statistical averages from the general population rather than ideal long-term health[27]. In a society where suboptimal health has become so common, "normal" does not always mean optimal. Often, it means common.

Many people begin experiencing symptoms long before laboratory values cross official thresholds for disease. Someone may be told their thyroid labs are "normal" while struggling with fatigue, brain fog, hair loss, constipation, or difficulty losing weight. Another person may technically remain within standard glucose ranges while insulin resistance continues advancing for years.

This does not mean laboratory testing is flawed. Quite the opposite. Laboratory testing offers extraordinary insight. However, conventional medicine has traditionally focused on identifying disease only after dysfunction has advanced to the point that clear diagnostic criteria are met.

Preventive and longevity-oriented medicine asks a different question entirely: Where are labs trending long before irreversible damage develops? And that shift in perspective changes the entire conversation.

The Metabolic Story Most People Never Hear

Few conditions illustrate the progression of hidden illness more clearly than metabolic strain. For many individuals, metabolic disease becomes synonymous with diabetes itself, but the process often begins years — or even decades — before blood sugar officially rises into diabetic ranges[28].

In the early stages of insulin resistance, the pancreas produces more insulin in an attempt to keep glucose appearing "normal[29]." From the outside, standard laboratory work may still look reassuring while important physiological changes are already unfolding internally.

During this stage, it is common to experience symptoms that are often dismissed as "life," such as:

- intense cravings
- constant hunger
- fatigue after meals
- energy crashes
- stubborn weight gain
- brain fog
- increasing abdominal fat
- dependence on frequent eating to maintain energy

This is one of the reasons fasting insulin became such an important marker for me clinically. By the time blood sugar finally rises enough to trigger a diagnosis of prediabetes or diabetes, the disease may already have been brewing for a very long time. And this is precisely why chronic diseases can feel so confusing and frustrating.

It is not uncommon for someone to spend years feeling progressively worse while repeatedly being told, 'Everything looks normal,' only to one day suddenly be diagnosed with diabetes as though it appeared out of nowhere.

This naturally leads patients to ask the same question: "Why did nobody tell me this earlier?" The answer is nuanced. Much of conventional medicine has historically focused on diagnosing disease once clear diagnostic thresholds are reached rather than identifying subtle dysfunction earlier in the process. Standard laboratory panels commonly include glucose, cholesterol, liver enzymes, kidney function, thyroid screening, and hemoglobin A1C — markers that often become abnormal later as dysfunction advances. But fasting insulin itself has not traditionally been emphasized as a routine screening marker in conventional medical settings. Yet elevated insulin may be one of the earliest warning signs the body gives us[30].

Part of this comes from medical training. Part comes from insurance reimbursement structures. And part of this stems from the fact that prevention-focused and longevity-oriented medicine are still relatively new models compared to the traditional disease-management framework that has shaped much of healthcare.

The Cardiometabolic Connection

A longstanding paradigm in healthcare is the tendency to separate the body into isolated compartments. Cardiovascular health, inflammation, metabolism, hormones, sleep, visceral fat, blood sugar regulation, stress, and muscle mass are deeply interconnected. The body tells one larger physiological story. Cardiovascular disease is one of the clearest examples of why this matters so profoundly.

Heart disease is widely perceived as a sudden event, but plaque formation and vascular dysfunction typically develop silently over long periods of time[31] while the body continues compensating.

Too often, the first symptom of cardiovascular disease is a heart attack. That reality completely changes the importance of looking earlier. Long before catastrophe occurs, prolonged physiological strains frequently leave biochemical clues[32]:

- rising triglycerides
- worsening glucose regulation
- elevated fasting insulin
- increasing visceral fat
- elevated blood pressure
- inflammatory markers such as hs-CRP
- fatty liver
- declining exercise capacity
- and slower recovery

One of the things that drew me so strongly toward longevity and preventive medicine was seeing how much opportunity exists before advanced disease fully develops. And yet, far too many individuals spend years focusing only on whether a single cholesterol number or A1C level falls within a standard range without understanding the much larger metabolic and inflammatory context surrounding it.

The Hidden Clues I Pay Attention To

Over the years, I have found certain laboratory markers especially valuable for interpreting physiology from a preventive and longevity-focused perspective. Laboratory values are not moral judgments, and no single number defines the health or worth of an entire human being. They are simply pieces of information that can help reveal patterns earlier, while there is still tremendous opportunity to support the body and potentially change direction. Some of the markers I pay particular close attention include:

Fasting Insulin

One of the earliest and most valuable indicators of health dysfunction. Insulin resistance often develops long before glucose becomes abnormal. I prefer to see fasting insulin around 2–6 uIU/mL.

Hemoglobin A1C

Although prediabetes officially begins at 5.7%, many preventive and longevity-focused practitioners prefer seeing A1C closer to 5.0-5.3%.

Triglycerides and HDL

These markers can offer valuable insight into health and insulin sensitivity when interpreted together. I prefer triglycerides below approximately 80 mg/dL and HDL above approximately 50 mg/dL in women and 40 mg/dL in men, while also paying close attention to the triglyceride-to-HDL ratio, since lower ratios are often associated with better insulin sensitivity and overall metabolic health.

ApoB and Lipoprotein(a)

These cardiovascular markers have become increasingly important in preventive cardiology because they provide far more meaningful insight into cardiovascular risk than total cholesterol alone. In general, I prefer ApoB below 80 mg/dL in most individuals focused on prevention, and even lower in higher-risk patients. Lipoprotein(a), or Lp(a), is more heavily influenced by genetics and can significantly increase long-term cardiovascular risk when elevated. Ideally, I prefer to see it below 30 mg/dL, but the lower, the better.

hs-CRP

An inflammatory marker that can sometimes reveal underlying stress and cardiovascular risk long before symptoms fully develop.

Thyroid Markers

TSH, Free T3, thyroid antibodies, and a broader thyroid evaluation can help explain fatigue, metabolic slowing, mood changes, cognitive symptoms, and shifts in energy regulation that may otherwise be overlooked.

Ferritin, Vitamin D, B12, and Folate

Nutrient deficiencies and suboptimal levels frequently contribute to fatigue, neurological symptoms, poor recovery, low resilience, and impaired function. In general, I like to see ferritin at least 50 ng/mL, depending on the individual context; vitamin D around 60–80 ng/mL; and B12 and folate within robust functional ranges rather than barely above deficiency thresholds. If your healthcare provider recommends iron supplementation, keep in mind that vitamin C may help improve iron absorption. Likewise, if vitamin D supplementation is recommended, adequate magnesium status is important because magnesium is involved in vitamin D activation and utilization.

Hormonal Markers

Estradiol, progesterone, testosterone, DHEA-S, SHBG, FSH, and LH often provide important insights into resilience, recovery, long-term health, aging, and overall adaptation. DHEA-S is a hormone produced primarily by the adrenal glands and can provide clues about stress adaptation and overall vitality. SHBG (sex hormone-binding globulin) is a protein that influences how much estrogen and testosterone are available for your body to use. FSH (follicle-stimulating hormone) and LH (luteinizing hormone) help regulate ovarian function and can provide valuable insights into reproductive health and the menopausal transition.

Data Without Fear

The danger of having access to so much data is that information can easily become anxiety-provoking. People begin obsessing over every laboratory fluctuation, every symptom, and every latest alarmist trend on social media.

But prevention was never meant to create fear. Its purpose is awareness. There is an enormous difference between those two states. Fear disconnects people from themselves. Awareness helps people respond more intentionally. When approached thoughtfully, laboratory work can be tremendously empowering because it allows people to recognize changes earlier, rather than waiting for advanced disease to force attention later.

With proper guidance, numbers stop being sources of shame and become tools for clarity. Ultimately, this is about understanding the body clearly enough to support it more intentionally, more compassionately, and earlier than previous generations ever did. If you only remember one thing from this chapter, let it be this: Labs reveal direction, not destiny.

Chapter 8

The Cost of Constant Stimulation

★★★

Almost everything will work again if
you unplug it for a few minutes, including you.
— Anne Lamott

A Nervous System on High Alert

By the time most people begin to question their energy, focus, stress levels, or sense of well-being, the nervous system has been repeating the same patterns for years. Constant stimulation, mental overload, and emotional pressure stopped feeling unusual because the body learned to function within those conditions.

The remarkable thing about the nervous system is that it is shaped by repetition. Whatever is experienced repeatedly begins to feel normal, even when it is not necessarily healthy. A heightened state of activation can become so customary that slowing down can feel strangely uncomfortable.

What makes this especially difficult to recognize is that modern life often rewards the very behaviors that keep the nervous system activated. Constant availability is mistaken for dedication. Busyness becomes a measure of importance. Productivity is celebrated while recovery is postponed. Over time, people begin assuming that feeling rushed, mentally crowded, or perpetually fatigued is part of adulthood rather than a signal that something deeper may need attention.

This is one of the reasons chronic stress can be difficult to recognize. The body learns to accommodate it, the mind learns to expect it, and life continues moving forward. From the outside, everything may appear functional. Yet internally, the nervous system may have been carrying a tremendous burden for far longer than it can truly handle.

Rest Was Never Meant to Feel Earned

Wellness culture tends to present health as though it belongs only to people capable of maintaining flawless routines and constant discipline. That image collapses quickly when confronted with real life. People are navigating demanding careers, financial pressure, family discord, emotional burden, caregiving responsibilities, and life circumstances that leave very little energy remaining for themselves by the end of the day. Under those conditions, consistency becomes difficult long before healing even begins.

A particularly damaging belief surrounding health is the idea that if someone cannot do everything correctly, there is little value in doing anything at all. As a result, rest becomes even more delayed. Slowing down becomes associated with laziness. Silence creates guilt instead of relief. Even moments of recovery begin feeling unproductive. But healing rarely begins through intensity. It begins the moment someone stops treating their body like a machine that must constantly perform without pause.

Healing often begins when life no longer feels relentlessly accelerated. It may start with something surprisingly simple: sitting outside for a few quiet minutes without reaching for a phone, lingering over a meal instead of rushing through it, or allowing bedtime to arrive without resisting it. Gradually, small moments of stillness begin returning to places where urgency once seemed to dominate everything. What at first feels unfamiliar slowly becomes a source of restoration. For some individuals, the real surprise is discovering that rest can exist without needing to be earned first.

Sleep Is Biological Repair

It is not uncommon to describe functioning on four or five hours of sleep as an admirable superhuman power, as though overriding basic biological needs reflects strength rather than depletion. Yet some of the most important restorative processes occur while we sleep.

During sleep, the brain clears accumulated waste products, consolidates memories, processes emotional experiences, and activates countless repair mechanisms[33]. Immune regulation, tissue repair, hormonal signaling, and metabolic recovery all depend on adequate sleep. Far from being passive inactivity, sleep is one of the most biologically active periods of the day.

The challenge is that the consequences of insufficient sleep rarely appear all at once. Instead, they gradually accumulate through changes in mood, concentration, appetite regulation, recovery, and metabolic health. Long before someone notices a problem, the body may already be paying the price.

In the book *Why We Sleep*, sleep researcher Matthew Walker describes a particularly concerning phenomenon: human beings gradually lose the ability to accurately recognize how impaired they have become under chronic sleep deprivation[34]. That insight explains why exhaustion often becomes accepted long before people fully appreciate its impact on mood, concentration, hunger, emotional steadiness, decision-making, or long-term health.

Current research consistently suggests that most adults require approximately seven to nine hours of sleep per night for proper restoration and long-term health[35]. Yet large portions of the population sleep far less, assuming the body will adapt without consequence.

The problem is that adaptation does not mean absence of impact. Research has repeatedly linked chronic sleep deprivation to increased cardiovascular risk, impaired blood sugar regulation, and even higher rates of cognitive decline later in life, including Alzheimer's disease[36,37]. In other words, insufficient sleep affects far more than just energy levels.

Breathing Shapes Internal State

Breathing occupies a unique place in human biology because it operates both automatically and voluntarily. It continues without conscious effort, yet it can also be consciously regulated within seconds. Few bodily functions influence both mind and body so directly.

In *Breath*, James Nestor explores the counterintuitive idea that we breathe far more often and more shallowly than our bodies require[38]. Chronic overbreathing, especially through the mouth, has been associated with heightened internal stress, poor sleep quality, reduced carbon dioxide tolerance, and greater nervous system activation. In other words, the way people breathe throughout the day may subtly reinforce the same internal urgency they are trying to escape.

One of the most surprising observations I have made over the years is how rarely people experience moments of genuine presence. Meals are often eaten while scrolling through a phone, driving, answering messages, watching television, planning the next task, or mentally replaying the previous one. Attention becomes so divided that many people move through entire days without fully noticing the experience of being where they are.

This became especially apparent when I began encouraging people to pause briefly before meals or at different points throughout the day and take several slow breaths. The suggestion seemed almost too simple to matter. Yet the responses were unexpectedly emotional. Several people later shared that they could not remember the last time they had eaten without simultaneously multitasking or feeling mentally preoccupied. A few intentional breaths created enough space for presence to reappear.

One simple technique I frequently recommend is box breathing, a structured breathing exercise commonly used in stress-regulation practices. The process is straightforward: inhale slowly for four seconds, hold the breath for four seconds, exhale for four seconds, then pause again for four seconds before repeating the cycle. The power of this exercise lies not in complexity, but in the repeated act of deliberately slowing the breath. This simple shift can begin to signal safety to the nervous system, helping to interrupt the constant internal urgency.

While writing this book, I found myself returning to this technique repeatedly. The process of organizing ideas, revising chapters, and communicating meaningful concepts can become unexpectedly activating. Pausing for a few slow, structured breaths repeatedly helped bring my attention back into the present moment while calming my nervous system. It is extraordinary how quickly the body can respond to small actions whose impact is easy to underestimate.

Attention Has Become Fragmented

Modern life competes aggressively for our attention. Previous generations experienced silence far more regularly than most people do today. Empty moments occurred naturally throughout the day, often without ubiquitous digital interruptions immediately filling every pause.

Today, even brief moments of stillness tend to disappear almost immediately because we have become accustomed to reaching for stimulation whenever space appears. Many individuals rarely remain alone with their thoughts long enough to notice their minds fully settling.

Attention itself becomes fragmented, reflection shortens, presence weakens, and quiet begins to feel uncomfortable as the brain adapts to continuous input. Even rest can become mentally crowded. Someone may sit down at the end of the day, believing they are relaxing, while the mind continues absorbing stimulation from multiple directions simultaneously. The body remains physically still, yet internally the nervous system never fully settles. This constant turmoil distances people from the experience of inner stillness.

This is one of the reasons practices such as meditation have become increasingly valuable for many individuals. At its core, meditation is not about “stopping thoughts” or achieving some perfect state of calm. It is the practice of learning to sit with attention more intentionally again, rather than being endlessly pulled outward by stimulation, distraction, and mental noise.

In its simplest form, meditation may involve nothing more than sitting quietly for a few minutes and focusing on the breath. Thoughts will almost certainly arise. Plans, worries, memories, distractions, and mental commentary tend to appear almost immediately. Just notice the thoughts without becoming carried away by them. Each time attention drifts, gently return to the breath or the present moment. Truthfully, the practice of meditation is less about achieving silence and more about repeatedly returning to awareness. Even brief moments of intentional stillness can begin to change people's relationship with their own minds.

Returning to Life Again

As people begin incorporating some of these practices more intentionally into daily life, prioritizing sleep, slowing the breath, creating moments of quiet, and reducing constant stimulation, the internal experience of life begins to change in ways that are initially subtle yet meaningful. The shifts often emerge through ordinary moments that begin to feel different. The mind settles more easily, rest becomes more restorative, and conversations feel more present. Silence no longer creates the same discomfort it once did. Little by little, the body stops responding as though urgency is constantly required for survival. What changes most profoundly is often invisible from the outside. Life begins to feel less like something that must be managed constantly and more like something that can be experienced as it unfolds.

The goal is not to become a different person, eliminate every source of stress, or achieve a permanent state of calm. Rather, it is the gradual recognition that many of the qualities people seek—greater clarity, emotional steadiness, resilience, and presence—emerge naturally when the nervous system is given opportunities to rest, recover, and feel safe again. In that sense, healing often involves returning to parts of yourself that had been quietly buried beneath years of constant stimulation.

Many of the practices that support this shift are not new. For thousands of years, people have understood the value of stillness, rest, reflection, connection, and time in nature. Life eventually became loud enough to pull us away from them. Perhaps part of restoration involves remembering what we knew long before modern life convinced us to forget.

Chapter 9

Living in a Toxic World

★★★

The dose makes the poison.
— Paracelsus

The Ice Cube Trays

A whole encyclopedia could be written about toxins. They are present in the air we breathe, the water we drink, the products around our homes, the packaging that touches our food, and numerous other parts of daily life. Trying to eliminate every possible exposure would become unsustainable.

That is not the purpose of this chapter. Rather, the focus is awareness. More specifically, learning to recognize some of the simplest opportunities to reduce unnecessary burden in ways that feel realistic and manageable in everyday life.

Ironically, one of the moments that brought this into focus for me happened in my own kitchen. As I was preparing educational material for patients about reducing toxins, I walked to my freezer to grab ice. It struck me that I had been using the same inexpensive plastic ice cube trays from the dollar store for years. I had probably filled them and reused them thousands of times without ever questioning them for a second. I remember laughing at the irony. Here I was teaching others about reducing environmental toxins while simultaneously overlooking something sitting directly in front of me every single day.

The experience reminded me how easily routine can make even obvious things invisible. Even as we become more health-conscious, we continue to discover blind spots. None of us sees everything clearly all the time. Not every product or environment needs to be viewed as dangerous. It is about becoming a little more intentional, making small changes feel realistic and manageable.

Why Toxins Matter

These exposures matter because many of the chemicals encountered may function as endocrine disruptors[39]. In practical terms, this means certain environmental substances may interfere with the same hormonal systems involved in fertility, metabolism, thyroid function, mood regulation, growth, and numerous processes that help the body maintain internal balance.

What makes this relevant is not necessarily a single exposure, but repetition. Over time, the body is asked to continuously recognize, process, filter, neutralize, and eliminate many harmful substances while simultaneously maintaining internal balance. So, even if occasional exposure does not automatically cause harm, repetition matters far more than we were ever taught to consider. And because eliminating toxins from our lives is unrealistic, a more balanced approach is to be more intentional about the exposures we can consistently reduce.

Plastics Everywhere

Reducing the chemical burden often begins with the materials that surround food and water. Disposable bottles, takeout packaging, food storage containers, utensils, and synthetic packaging materials have become so ubiquitous that most people rarely stop to question them.

One of the easiest places to begin is with food storage. Glass containers allow leftovers and prepared meals to be stored without food coming into direct contact with synthetic surfaces. Even when the lids still contain plastic components, reducing direct food contact itself may still be beneficial. No one needs to replace everything at once. But little by little, moving away from synthetic food containers may significantly lower chemical contact.

Heat deserves particular attention in these conversations. Placing hot food into takeout containers, reheating meals in synthetic storage containers, or microwaving food in disposable packaging may increase chemical migration into food[40]. Whenever possible, transferring meals into a glass before reheating is one of the simplest adjustments to implement.

Water creates another important conversation because hydration is something everyone requires daily. In many cities, tap water may contain varying levels of contaminants such as microplastics, pesticide residues, industrial chemicals, heavy metals, chlorine byproducts, and even traces of pharmaceuticals[41]. Because of this, it is understandable that many turn toward bottled water, believing it to be the healthier option. Used occasionally during travel or situations where convenience is necessary, is sometimes unavoidable. But relying heavily on disposable plastic bottles every day creates another form of repeated contact with the packaging, particularly when bottles are exposed to heat during storage and transportation.

For that reason, one of my favorite long-term investments for households is a reverse osmosis water filtration system. While the initial cost may seem high, many systems last for years with only periodic filter replacements. Over time, the cost becomes comparable to, and sometimes even lower than, the cost of continuously purchasing bottled water. More importantly, it allows families to reduce both water contaminants and unnecessary dependence on disposable bottles. Reusable glass or stainless-steel containers can then become standard household practices.

I sometimes think about how many years my own children drank water and milk from plastic cups and ate from plastic plates. Like many parents, I chose them because they were practical. They did not break when dropped, they were easy to clean, and they seemed perfectly safe. That experience reminds me how difficult it can be to recognize exposures that have become normal. Most people are not consciously choosing to increase their chemical burden. They are living within the environment and the information available to them at the time, just as I was.

One finding from recent research felt difficult to ignore. A study conducted at the University of New Mexico analyzed human brain tissue collected from autopsies and identified a measurable accumulation of microplastics in the brain. Researchers estimated that in some individuals, the amount identified roughly corresponded to the volume of a small plastic spoon[42]. Whether future research ultimately confirms the full significance of those findings remains to be seen, but the observation alone is difficult to ignore. It is one thing to think about plastics as part of the environment around us. It is another thing to imagine them accumulating inside our tissues.

Fragrances, and the Air We Live In

Fragrances are among the most overlooked sources of chemical exposure. Perfumes, scented candles, plug-in air fresheners, laundry products, room sprays, and many fragranced household items release synthetic compounds into indoor air continuously throughout the day[43]. Many of these products emit volatile organic compounds (VOCs), a diverse group of airborne chemicals that can contribute to indoor air pollution and, over time, increase the body's overall chemical burden. Yet because pleasant scents have become so strongly associated with cleanliness, comfort, and even self-care, these everyday sources rarely receive much attention.

This does not mean you must suddenly throw away every perfume bottle you own. But you may choose to gradually reduce daily fragrance use by improving ventilation, using perfumes more lightly, or replacing certain products with simpler alternatives. As with many other aspects of this chapter, the intention is not to alarm. It is simply becoming more conscious of the environments we repeatedly create around ourselves.

Cleaning Products and Everyday Contact

Cleaning products are another area where simple changes can help reduce repeated exposure to harsh cleaning agents. Conventional household cleaners contain compounds that stay present on surfaces we touch daily. Yet for basic household cleaning, simpler alternatives are highly effective. Vinegar, baking soda, castile soap, and fragrance-free products can handle far more than most people expect.

Even thermal paper receipts deserve a brief mention. Many receipts contain compounds such as BPA and similar chemicals that may be absorbed through skin contact[44]. Saying "no receipt" when possible, or minimizing unnecessary handling, is a small, simple way to reduce exposure.

What We Put on the Body

Personal care products deserve attention, too, because the skin absorbs far more than is commonly acknowledged. Deodorants, lotions, cosmetics, shampoos, and skincare products may contain long lists of chemicals most people never pay attention to. This does not mean every product must suddenly become "clean" overnight. But being more selective over time matters.

I personally stopped using conventional deodorant regularly because I became increasingly concerned about applying heavily fragranced and chemically formulated products so close to breast tissue every single day. Instead, I began making a very simple alternative using organic coconut oil, baking soda, and a small amount of essential oil for fragrance. It does not work perfectly in every situation, especially during extreme heat or intense sweating, and it may not work for everyone. But for me, it became one simple way to reduce unnecessary chemical exposure.

Food by Design

Another important part of this conversation involves the food itself. Beyond excess sugar and highly refined oils, many modern packaged foods now contain long lists of artificial colors, flavor enhancers, preservatives, stabilizers, emulsifiers, sweeteners, and synthetic additives designed to intensify flavor, extend shelf life, improve texture, or make products more visually appealing.

Even terms that sound reassuring, such as "natural flavors," often refer to highly processed compounds produced in industrial food systems, far removed from anything that occurs in nature[45]. One of the simplest ways to think about this is to ask a very basic question: Would your great-grandparents have recognized these ingredients as food? Because the further a product moves from traditional ingredients, the more worthwhile it becomes to pause before making it part of daily life.

For most of history, food consisted of ingredients people could identify directly: they either grew from soil or they had a mother. Today, many products contain ingredient lists filled with substances most people cannot even pronounce. At some point, many foods stopped being food and became highly industrialized products, especially those marketed to children.

The question is not whether these toxins are allowed in food. The deeper question is what happens when the body, especially a child's developing body, is exposed to them repeatedly. Research has linked certain artificial colors and preservatives with increased hyperactivity in some children[46]. At the same time, other food additives, including emulsifiers commonly used to improve texture and shelf life, are being studied for their effects on the gut microbiome and intestinal barrier[47],[48].

That matters because food is not only fuel. It is material the body must identify, process, interpret, absorb, store, and respond to every single day. When foods become heavily industrialized formulations rather than simple ingredients, the body is asked to process substances it was never designed to encounter.

Awareness Without Obsession

The most important lesson toxins have taught me is that awareness and fear are not the same thing. Trying to eliminate every possible exposure from our lives would quickly become exhausting and unrealistic. We cannot avoid every synthetic compound, nor do we need to, to make meaningful changes. The most impactful shifts are also the simplest ones, repeated consistently over time.

This subject becomes easier to understand through the lens of automatic behaviors. Most daily habits exist precisely because they allow life to function automatically. We prepare food, store leftovers, clean the house, light candles, spray fragrances, drink water, heat meals, buy snacks, and move through our days without needing to consciously analyze every small decision repeatedly. The challenge is that many of these routines may also lead to repeated contact with substances we rarely question. What if we occasionally paused and asked the question: Which daily habits in my life have become so automatic that I no longer question them?

For one of my friends, it was realizing that her coffee maker dripped boiling water through plastic components every single morning. For me, it was something as simple as a pair of plastic ice cube trays sitting in my freezer for years without a second thought. Likely, everyone has their own version of the coffee maker or the ice cube trays story.

Chapter 10

28-Day Metabolic Restoration

★★★

The journey of a thousand miles begins with a single step.
— Lao Tzu

From Understanding to Action

Over the past several chapters, we have explored many of the factors that influence metabolic health. We have discussed sugar, ultra-processed foods, movement, sleep, stress, toxins, muscle, prevention, and the countless ways modern life can gradually pull the body away from its natural state of balance.

Understanding these concepts is important. Knowledge creates awareness, helping us recognize patterns that may have gone unnoticed for years. Yet information alone rarely changes health. Transformation occurs when knowledge becomes action. This is where structure becomes incredibly helpful.

Permanent lifestyle modifications can feel overwhelming. The idea of changing everything forever can create enough resistance to prevent any change from happening at all. A shorter period of focused effort often feels far more manageable. There is a beginning, a clear plan, and a defined endpoint.

The ***28-Day Metabolic Restoration*** (also known as the 28-MR) is a timed program that offers an opportunity to step outside routines and temporarily experience something different. Rather than wondering whether healthier habits might make a difference, you can see for yourself what your body can do when properly supported.

Throughout this chapter, you will learn the principles that guide this program. In Appendix C, you will also find a collection of recipes designed to help you apply these concepts in everyday life.

During this journey, some days will feel easier than others. You may encounter food urges, social situations, busy schedules, travel, unexpected setbacks, or moments when old habits feel difficult to break. None of those represent failure; they are simply part of the process.

Before continuing, I encourage you to complete the Pre-Program Metabolic Assessment in Appendix A if you have not already. The questionnaire will help you establish a baseline and identify symptoms that may have become so ever-present that they have faded into the background of daily life.

You may be surprised by how much can change in four weeks. More importantly, you may notice that many of the health improvements you have been seeking are connected in ways that are not always obvious. When the body begins moving toward better metabolic health, multiple bodily systems improve together.

What you are about to do is something special. For the next four weeks, you are choosing to place your health, energy, and well-being at the forefront of your priorities in a way that many people rarely do. You are stepping outside the momentum of everyday life and creating space for an experience that may once have felt out of reach.

Previous attempts might have left you discouraged. Or perhaps no one has ever provided the structure needed to make the process feel achievable. Whatever brings you here, now is the time.

The next four weeks offer you a unique opportunity. It is a chance to learn, experiment, and experience firsthand how your body responds when given the conditions it needs to thrive.

Let's begin.

The Seven Metabolic Restoration Commitments

The seven commitments are designed to focus your attention on simple core behaviors that influence multiple aspects of health simultaneously.

Commitment 1: Eat Real Food

Throughout the 28-MR, the emphasis shifts away from highly processed products and toward simple, recognizable ingredients. You will focus on foods that are as close as possible to their natural state.

Commitment 2: Eliminate Gluten

This recommendation provides an opportunity to temporarily remove a common dietary irritant and observe how your body responds. In addition, removing gluten often leads to a significant reduction in many refined, highly processed carbohydrate foods that dominate our diets. As a result, this commitment frequently influences far more than just gluten exposure.

Commitment 3: Keep Added Sugar Off Your Plate

Few dietary changes have the potential to influence metabolic health as quickly as reducing excess sugar. For the next four weeks, added sugar will be limited to no more than 20 grams per day; this does not include naturally occurring sugar found in foods such as fruit.

Commitment 4: Build Every Meal Around Protein

Protein becomes the anchor of every meal. Rather than viewing protein as an afterthought, begin with it first. This strategy helps promote muscle conservation, satiety, and blood sugar stability.

Commitment 5: Move Daily and Strengthen Twice Per Week

We are designed to move, but movement need not be extreme. Walking, cycling, swimming, yoga, Pilates, and other activities can all contribute to better health. The goal is consistency rather than intensity. In addition, aim to include at least two strength-training sessions each week to maintain muscle and long-term metabolic health.

Commitment 6: Protect Sleep

Many people view sleep as something that happens after everything else is finished. However, the body performs many of its most important restorative functions while we sleep. Protecting sleep may be one of the most powerful health interventions available. During the 28-MR, make a conscious effort to prioritize sleep and aim for at least seven hours of actual sleep each night. Begin treating sleep as a priority rather than an afterthought. Small improvements in sleep lead to meaningful gains in energy, appetite regulation, mood, and overall health.

Commitment 7: Prepare for Success

The most important commitment of all is preparation. Most people do not abandon healthy habits because they lack motivation. They struggle because life becomes busy, unexpected situations arise, and healthy choices become difficult to access in the moment. Planning ahead, keeping nutritious foods available, preparing meals, and reducing unnecessary friction considerably increase the likelihood of success.

None of these commitments is individually revolutionary. Their power comes from practicing them together and consistently. Think of them as the pillars supporting the entire framework. Every recommendation in the pages that follow will connect back to one or more of them. For now, you do not need to master everything at once. Just aim at becoming comfortable with the material.

Building Your Metabolic Restoration Kitchen

Success over the next 28 days will depend far less on willpower than on the systems you put in place. Many health decisions are made long before hunger appears. They are influenced by what is available in the refrigerator, what foods are visible in the pantry, what ingredients are easy to prepare, and what options are within reach when life gets busy.

This is why one of the most important steps occurs before Day One begins. Your kitchen is about to become a ***Metabolic Restoration Kitchen***. The goal is simple: create an environment that makes healthier choices easier. When the foods that align with your goals are readily available, making good decisions requires far less effort. If you're wondering exactly what I keep in my own kitchen, I've included Appendix D, "Your Metabolic Restoration Kitchen." There you'll find the pantry staples, refrigerator and freezer essentials, basic kitchen tools, and everyday ingredients I rely on most often. Think of it as a practical guide to stocking your kitchen to make healthy eating easier, one meal at a time.

Protein Becomes the Foundation

One of the simplest ways to prepare for success is to ensure that several protein options are always available. Eggs, poultry, seafood, beef, Greek yogurt, cottage cheese, and other high-quality protein sources can all serve as the foundation of a meal.

Personally, I find it incredibly helpful to make a single trip to a warehouse club such as Costco or Sam's Club and stock up on several different protein sources at once. Fish, chicken, shrimp, ground beef, eggs, and other protein-rich foods can be portioned into individual servings and stored in the freezer for later use. By keeping a variety of proteins readily available, I always know that the building blocks of a healthy meal are within reach. Having several options available makes home-cooked meals easier to prepare, reduces the temptation to rely on convenience foods, restaurant meals, or last-minute food decisions. It is also far less expensive than eating out regularly.

How Much Protein?

A common question people ask is how much protein they should eat. While individual needs vary, experts in muscle-centric medicine recommend approximately 1.5 to 2.2 grams of protein per kilogram of ideal body weight daily to maintain muscle health, metabolic function, and healthy aging[49]. For some readers, that amount may seem surprisingly high because many people consume far less protein than they realize, particularly at breakfast. Rather than becoming overly focused on exact calculations, focus on the bigger picture. Over the next 28 days, make a conscious effort to increase your protein intake and ensure that every meal includes a meaningful source of protein.

Whenever possible, choose higher-quality options such as pasture-raised eggs, grass-fed beef, organic poultry, or wild-caught seafood.

A Note for Vegetarians and Vegans

You may have noticed that the protein recommendations throughout this program emphasize animal-based protein sources. That is intentional. The nutritional approach used in the 28-Day Metabolic Restoration was designed around high-quality animal proteins for their nutrient density and amino acid profiles.

If you follow a vegetarian or vegan diet, I hope you'll continue reading with an open mind. While some of the specific dietary recommendations may not align with your personal choices, many of the principles explored throughout this book—including prioritizing whole foods, minimizing ultra-processed products, improving sleep, managing stress, increasing physical activity, and building sustainable daily habits—can support better metabolic health regardless of the way you choose to eat. My hope is that you'll find ideas you can adapt to your own lifestyle while continuing to make choices that reflect your values and personal preferences.

Vegetables Become the Default

Once protein is established, vegetables become the next priority. Broccoli, asparagus, zucchini, leafy greens, cucumbers, peppers, cauliflower, Brussels sprouts, green beans, and many other vegetables provide nutrients, fiber, and variety to meals while contributing to overall metabolic health. Choose several options you genuinely enjoy and keep them readily accessible in your kitchen. Whenever possible, wash, chop, cook, and store vegetables in a visible location. Foods that are easy to access are far more likely to be eaten.

Healthy Fats become a Staple

Healthy fats play an important role throughout the 28-MR. Extra-virgin olive oil, butter, avocados, olives, nuts, seeds, and other minimally processed fat sources can help increase satiety and make meals more flavorful. As you build your Metabolic Restoration Kitchen, make sure these foods are readily available. Keep extra-virgin olive oil in the pantry, avocados on the counter, nuts and seeds within reach, and other healthy fat sources stocked and ready to use. I recommend avoiding industrial seed oils, often referred to as vegetable oils. Common examples include soybean, corn, cottonseed, canola, or sunflower oil. These oils are found in many packaged foods, restaurant meals, salad dressings, sauces, and fried foods. They are typically manufactured using intensive industrial processing methods and are highly inflammatory.

What Needs to Be Removed from Your Kitchen

Building a Metabolic Restoration Kitchen is not only about adding healthier foods. It is also about reducing the visibility and accessibility of foods that may make the challenge more difficult. Before Day One, take some time to look through your pantry, refrigerator, freezer, countertops, and drawers. Foods containing gluten, sugary beverages, highly processed snack foods, and products with significant added sugar should be removed from your immediate environment whenever possible. This does not mean throwing everything away. Some people choose to donate unopened items. Others place them in a box and store them out of sight until the challenge is complete. The objective is simple: Do not place yourself in a situation where temptation is constantly sitting on the kitchen counter or staring at you every time you open a cabinet. Rather than focusing on everything being removed, focus on the space you are creating for foods that better promote your health.

The Metabolic Restoration Filter

No food list can cover every product, ingredient, restaurant meal, or situation you will encounter. Eventually, you need something more useful than memorization. You need a way to think. That is the value of the ***Metabolic Restoration Filter.***

The Seven Metabolic Restoration Commitments that we discussed earlier provide the basis of the program. They establish the behaviors that improve metabolic health throughout the next four weeks. Yet, when you are standing in a grocery store aisle, looking at a restaurant menu, or deciding whether a particular food belongs on your plate, you need something more practical than a list of commitments. You need a quick decision-making tool. Think of the commitments as the overall strategy and the Metabolic Restoration filters as the day-to-day tool that helps you apply that strategy in real life. When you are unsure whether a food aligns with the program, ask the following four questions.

Question 1: Did it come from a plant or an animal?

This is the real-food question. Most of the foods that support health are remarkably simple. Vegetables, fruit, nuts, seeds, eggs, seafood, poultry, and meat all share something in common: they were grown, harvested, raised, or caught. This question encourages you to pause and consider where food comes from. The closer it remains to its natural origin, the more likely it is to advance your metabolic efforts. When a product is difficult to trace to a plant or animal, or has been heavily altered from its original form, it is worth taking a closer look before adding it to your diet.

Question 2: Is it gluten-free?

During these 28 days, gluten is removed completely. This means avoiding wheat, barley, rye, and foods made from them, including most breads, pasta, crackers, pastries, flour tortillas, and many packaged products unless clearly labeled gluten-free. Removing gluten temporarily allows you to see how your body responds in its absence. Over the past several decades, wheat-based foods have become a major part of our diet, and we tend to consume them multiple times per day without giving them much thought. At the same time, digestive complaints, food sensitivities, and other inflammatory conditions have become increasingly common. While gluten is not necessarily problematic for everyone, many individuals are surprised by how different they feel after removing it for a period of time. Take note of how you feel and let your own experience guide your conclusions.

Question 3: Does it contain little or no added sugar?
The target is no more than 20 grams of added sugar per day. One reason added sugar deserves special consideration is that it accumulates quickly. A flavored yogurt here, a granola bar there, a sweetened coffee drink, and suddenly, you have already consumed far more added sugar than you realized. When reading a label, look specifically at the "Added Sugars" section. If a single serving contains more than 5–10 grams of added sugar, it will quickly use a substantial portion of your daily allowance.

Question 4: Is it minimally processed?
This question helps you look beyond marketing claims. A food may come from a plant or animal, be gluten-free, and contain little or no added sugar, yet still be highly processed. The ingredient list often tells a more complete story than the front of the package. If a product contains ingredients you would not commonly have in your own kitchen, artificial colors, flavor enhancers, preservatives, emulsifiers, artificial sweeteners, or a long list of unfamiliar compounds, pause before making it part of your diet. The simpler and more recognizable the ingredient list, the more likely it is to fit with the 28-Day Metabolic Restoration.

These four questions are meant to create clarity, to help you make better decisions with greater confidence and consistency. A food does not need to be perfect to have a place in your diet, but the foundation of your meals should come from foods that pass the filter easily.

There is also an important distinction between core foods and enhancement foods. Core foods make up most of your meals: protein, vegetables, and healthy fats. These should pass the filter most of the time. Enhancement foods are small additions that make healthy meals more enjoyable, such as dressings, sauces, marinades, seasonings, or condiments. Some enhancement foods may not pass every part of the filter, but they can still have a place when used thoughtfully and in small amounts. For example, a flavored glaze or dressing may contain a few grams of added sugar or a less-than-ideal ingredient. But if a small amount helps you enjoy a large salad with protein, vegetables, and extra-virgin olive oil, it may still support the broader objective. The overall quality of the meal matters far more than the perfection of any single ingredient.

Meal Architecture

Although nutrition and architecture may appear to have little in common, they share an important principle. Strong structures are not built by accident. Before the first wall is raised, before the first window is installed, and long before the building becomes visible, there is a blueprint that provides organization. It allows individual pieces to work together as part of a larger whole. Nutrition is no different.

One reason people feel disoriented about food is that they focus on individual ingredients while losing sight of how the meal fits together. One day, the focus is on carbohydrates. Another day, it is calories. Then sugar or fat, then protein. ***Meal Architecture*** is a way of bringing the whole picture back into focus. Rather than thinking of food as a collection of individual choices, it encourages you to view meals as intentionally designed systems.

Once the meal-building method is established, decisions become much easier. Instead of constantly asking what to eat, you begin focusing on how to build a meal. Additionally, as your palate adapts and your body begins to respond differently, foods that once felt restrictive or unappealing often become ones you look forward to eating.

The Blueprint

Every meal in the 28-Day Metabolic Restoration follows the same basic blueprint:

- ✓ First, choose a protein source
- ✓ Next, add vegetables
- ✓ Third, add healthy fats

Once those three pieces are in place, the foundation of the meal is complete. Depending on your goals, activity level, preferences, and stage of the challenge, additional foods may be added, but the blueprint remains the same. When these components work together, meals become easier to build, more satisfying, and more conducive to metabolic health.

The beauty of Meal Architecture is that it provides consistency without requiring rigid meal plans or complicated rules. The specific foods may change from one meal to the next, but the underlying pattern remains substantially similar.

Meal Architecture in Action

The easiest way to understand Meal Architecture is to see it in practice. Notice that each meal looks different, yet the same foundational formula applies. Rather than memorizing specific recipes, focus on recognizing the blueprint. Once you understand the structure, you can create a wide variety of meals that support your health while still reflecting your personal preferences and lifestyle.

Breakfast:	Protein: Eggs Vegetables: Spinach, peppers, onions Healthy Fat: Avocado
Lunch:	Protein: Grilled chicken Vegetables: Large mixed salad Healthy Fat: Extra-virgin olive oil
Dinner:	Protein: Salmon Vegetables: Asparagus or zucchini Healthy Fat: Butter or olive oil

The Finishing Touches

Once the foundation is in place, there is room for additional foods that add variety, enjoyment, and flexibility to meals. Examples include fruit, sweet potatoes, white potatoes, rice, quinoa, and, later in the challenge, beans and legumes. These foods can absolutely be part of a healthy diet. Within the Meal Architecture framework, they are additions to the meal rather than the meal itself. This distinction matters because many people are accustomed to building meals around starches and treating protein as an afterthought. A plate of pasta with a small amount of chicken, a large serving of rice with a few bites of meat, pizza, or a baked potato that becomes the centerpiece of the meal are common examples. Meal Architecture reverses that pattern. Think of these foods the same way an architect thinks about finishing touches in a home. They add character, variety, and personalization, but they are not what holds the meal together.

If all of this still feels somewhat abstract, do not worry. In Appendix C, you will find a collection of breakfast, lunch, and dinner recipes that demonstrate these principles in practice.

Week One: Reset and Simplify

Now that we have explored the framework and established the principles that will guide this program, it is time to begin the actual 28-Day Metabolic Restoration (28-MR). The next four weeks are where knowledge becomes action.

Week One is the most challenging but also the most important. For many participants, this will be the first time in years they have intentionally stepped away from processed foods, excess sugar, and the constant stream of highly engineered products that dominate the modern food environment. It is normal for the opening days to feel different.

Some people notice the intensity of their cravings. Others experience changes in energy, hunger, digestion, or mood. Some feel surprisingly good within a few days, while others require more time to adjust. Regardless of how your unique experience evolves, return to the core principles of the program whenever you feel uncertain about what to do:

1. Use the Metabolic Restoration Filter
2. Follow the blueprint of Meal Architecture
3. Keep added sugar below 20 grams per day
4. Remove gluten completely
5. Remove dairy during Week One
6. Remove beans and legumes until Week 3
7. Move your body daily (as discussed in Chapter 6)
8. Prioritize sleep (as discussed in Chapter 8)
9. Prepare your environment for success

You do not need to count calories, measure food, or create elaborate meal plans. Week One is about establishing a new rhythm and allowing your body to begin adapting to a different set of inputs. Trust the process, focus on consistency, and concentrate on completing the first seven days.

Why Is Dairy Removed During Week One?

Dairy is temporarily removed as part of the simplification process. This is not because dairy is inherently unhealthy. In fact, many dairy foods can be excellent sources of protein and other nutrients. Like gluten, dairy is a commonly consumed food group and can be difficult to evaluate when it is part of the diet every day. Temporarily removing it creates a chance to notice how your body responds. Some individuals have varying degrees of dairy intolerance or sensitivity without realizing it. For some people, removing dairy makes no difference. Others may experience improvements in digestion, bloating, congestion, skin symptoms, or overall comfort. The only way to know how your body reacts is to create a period of separation. Dairy will be reintroduced during Week Two, allowing you to evaluate it more intentionally and make decisions based on your own experience rather than assumptions.

Hydration Matters More Than You Think

Hydration is a simple but important part of caring for your body during the 28-Day Metabolic Restoration. A practical way to estimate your daily fluid needs is to aim for approximately half your body weight in ounces of fluids each day. For example, a person weighing 150 pounds would aim for about 75 ounces daily (approximately 2 to 3 liters). This is not a rigid rule, but rather a helpful starting point that can be adjusted based on climate, activity level, and individual needs.

Hydration can include plain water, mineral water, herbal teas, and clean electrolyte beverages. Electrolytes may be particularly helpful for individuals who exercise regularly, sweat heavily, live in hot climates, or experience headaches, fatigue, or low energy during the 28-MR. When choosing an electrolyte product, look for options with little or no added sugar and minimal artificial ingredients. BodyBio E-Lyte and LyteShow are examples of products that align well with these principles.

You can also benefit from consuming apple cider vinegar. While not required, this simple practice may increase feelings of fullness and moderate post-meal glucose responses in some individuals. If you choose to use apple cider vinegar, select an organic version with "the mother" and start with 1 to 2 teaspoons diluted in a glass of water first thing in the morning or before a meal.

Finally, the quality of your water matters greatly. As discussed in Chapter 9, whenever possible, choose properly filtered water and store it in glass or stainless-steel containers rather than plastic ones. Hydration is one of the simplest habits in the entire program, yet it can have a surprisingly meaningful impact on how you feel.

What About Coffee?

You may be wondering whether coffee is allowed. The answer is yes. If you are a coffee drinker, one to two cups of coffee per day can fit comfortably within the 28-MR framework. In fact, coffee provides a useful opportunity to practice using the Metabolic Restoration Filter. Let's run it through the four questions together.

- ✓ Did it come from a plant or an animal? Yes.
- ✓ Is it gluten-free? Yes.
- ✓ Does it contain little or no added sugar? This is correct for black coffee. However, many popular coffee beverages contain significant amounts of added sugar through syrups, flavored creamers, and other sweetened ingredients.
- ✓ Is it minimally processed? Plain coffee generally is. Roasted and ground coffee beans remain a relatively simple food product. On the other hand, many specialty coffee drinks contain a long list of additives, flavorings, and highly processed ingredients.

As you can see, coffee itself is not usually the issue. More often, the problem lies in what gets added to it. If you prefer something in your coffee, keep it simple. As discussed in Chapter 5, allulose, stevia, and monk fruit are the sweeteners I recommend when used in their purest forms. For those who tolerate dairy, a small amount of heavy whipping cream can be an option. If dairy is not well tolerated or is being avoided during Week One, consider an unsweetened non-dairy alternative such as coconut, almond, or cashew milk. Whenever possible, choose products with the shortest ingredient list and the fewest additives.

What About Intermittent Fasting?

Intermittent fasting is not required for the 28-MR. The primary focus of this program is improving the quality of the foods you eat rather than restricting when you eat them. However, if you already practice intermittent fasting and feel well doing so, there is no reason to stop. Many individuals choose to eat within a shorter eating window and may skip breakfast as part of that approach.

Potential benefits of intermittent fasting include improved appetite regulation, metabolic flexibility, and periods of lower insulin exposure. At the same time, meal timing is only one piece of the metabolic health puzzle. Food quality remains the foundation. If you choose to eat only two meals per day, make sure those meals contain adequate protein, vegetables, fiber, and healthy fats. It is important to meet your nutritional needs regardless of how many meals you consume per day.

What About Snacks?

Ideally, your body should be able to move comfortably from one meal to the next without needing a snack. When meals are built using the principles of Meal Architecture and contain adequate protein, vegetables, and healthy fats, energy is more stable, there are less preoccupation with food, and less desire to eat between meals.

At the same time, it is important to recognize that many of us have spent years relying on frequent snacking. During the first week, it is completely normal for old habits to surface. Before reaching for a snack, pause for a moment and consider whether you may be thirsty. Sometimes what feels like hunger is actually a need for hydration. Try drinking a glass of water and give your body a few minutes to adjust. Going for a short walk, stepping away from the kitchen, or redirecting your attention for a few minutes can also help you determine whether you are truly hungry or simply responding out of habit.

If you are still genuinely hungry, do not force yourself to wait until the next meal. Instead, choose a simple whole-food option that aligns with the program. Whenever possible, think of snacks as mini-meals rather than times to eat processed convenience foods. Here are some 28-MR snack examples:

- A hard-boiled egg
- A handful of minimally processed nuts
- Celery sticks or an apple with natural peanut butter or almond butter
- Sliced cucumbers, or bell peppers with guacamole
- A small bowl of berries with a handful of nuts
- Olives
- Avocado with a pinch of sea salt
- A few slices of turkey rolled around cucumber strips
- Leftover vegetables drizzled with extra-virgin olive oil

Common Week One Challenges

Cravings are common during the first week and are driven as much by habit as by physical hunger. Give yourself time to adjust and remember that lasting change takes practice.

Social situations often become the first real test. Family gatherings, restaurant meals, celebrations, and work events can present challenges. Rather than focusing on what you cannot control, focus on making the best choice available in the moment.

Headaches, fatigue, brain fog, irritability, or lightheadedness during the first few days of the program can be common. If this happens, do not be alarmed. Many people are surprised by these symptoms and mistakenly assume they are getting sick or that something is wrong. In most cases, these temporary symptoms reflect the body's adaptation to a different nutritional environment. Reducing processed foods, added sugars, and highly refined carbohydrates can influence fluid balance, electrolyte needs, appetite regulation, and energy metabolism. Staying well hydrated, using electrolytes when appropriate, prioritizing sleep, and eating adequate protein can make this transition more comfortable.

The good news is that these symptoms are usually short-lived and begin to improve within a few days as the body adjusts to its new routine.

One of the most important principles of the 28-MR is progress over perfection. Many people approach a program like this with an all-or-nothing mindset. They have one off-plan meal, one dessert, or one difficult day and immediately feel as though they have failed. Nothing could be further from the truth. One imperfect meal does not erase a week of good decisions, just as one healthy meal does not instantly transform your health. What matters most is the overall direction of your choices. If you find yourself off track, return to the plan at your next meal and keep moving forward.

Week Two: Build Momentum

By the second week, the initial adjustment period often settles. Cravings may be less intense, preparation may feel more natural, and the principles of Meal Architecture are no longer new. What required conscious effort during the first week may already feel more natural.

Week Two is about curiosity. Rather than strictly following the program, you become more attuned to your body's feedback. You will experiment and learn. For some individuals, changes may already be noticeable. For others, they may be more subtle. Either way, Week Two allows you to become a more careful observer.

Reintroduction of Dairy

This week marks the reintroduction of dairy, which was removed during Week One to experience how you feel without it. Now that dairy is gradually being reintroduced, you have a useful point of comparison. Take note of how you feel and any changes in digestion, bloating, congestion, skin symptoms, energy levels, or overall comfort. You might discover that dairy has little or no impact on how you feel. Or you might find that certain dairy products agree with you better than others.

If you determine that dairy is not a problem for you, there is no reason to avoid it; make sure that you always choose full-fat dairy products. On the other hand, if you notice symptoms returning, consider experimenting further. You may do well with fermented dairy products such as Greek yogurt or kefir, while feeling that milk, ice cream, or certain cheeses are more bothersome.

Discovering New Foods

One of the unexpected benefits of the 28-MR is that it will encourage you to explore foods you may never have considered before. Initially, you may focus on what is being removed and worry that your options will become limited. Yet something interesting may happen. As the challenge progresses, attention gradually shifts from restriction toward discovery.

Perhaps you try a vegetable you have never purchased before. Maybe you experiment with a different type of seafood, discover a new herb or spice, or learn to prepare a favorite food in a completely different way. Some participants discover fermented foods for the first time. Others realize they enjoy foods they had previously overlooked and that now become lifelong favorites.

A common observation during this stage is a change in palate. Foods that once seemed bland become more enjoyable, and natural flavors become easier to appreciate. At the same time, some highly processed foods that once felt irresistible begin to lose some of their appeal.

By the end of Week Two, the most important skill is not perfection but observation. As you reintroduce dairy, explore new foods, and continue practicing Meal Architecture, begin noticing patterns. Which meals leave you satisfied? Which foods affect your digestion, energy, appetite, mood, or sleep? You do not need to track every detail. Become more observant and allow your own experience to teach you.

Week Three: Personalize Your Experience

By the third week, something interesting begins to happen. The 28-MR is starting to feel less like a challenge. Many of the decisions that required effort during the first two weeks no longer demand the same degree of intentionality. You may find yourself automatically building meals around protein, vegetables, and healthy fats without even thinking about it.

You might even notice that you move through the grocery store differently than before. You may spend more time around the perimeter of the store, where fresh foods are typically located. Produce, seafood, meat, poultry, eggs, and other minimally processed foods begin to stand out more. The center aisles often take on a different role as well. Rather than drawing you toward the chips, cookies, snack foods, sugary beverages, and highly processed convenience products, they become a place to find enhancement ingredients such as extra-virgin olive oil, vinegar, spices, seasonings, canned seafood, nuts, seeds, and other foods that complement the foundation of your meals.

This shift may seem small, but it represents something much larger. You are no longer following a set of instructions. You are beginning to build a new identity—one that sees food differently, shops differently, and makes decisions with greater intention.

Reintroducing Beans and Legumes

Foods such as black beans, pinto beans, lentils, chickpeas, and other legumes have been part of traditional diets worldwide for centuries. These foods were intentionally removed during the first two weeks of the 28-MR. The reason is that the early stages were designed to create as much clarity as possible. By temporarily removing foods that can occasionally contribute to digestive symptoms in some individuals, it becomes easier to identify how your body responds when they are added back.

As with dairy, many people tolerate beans and legumes extremely well. Others may notice bloating, gas, or digestive discomfort, particularly if they are not accustomed to eating them regularly. If you choose to reintroduce beans and legumes, start with modest portions and pay attention to your body's feedback.

It is also important to remember that beans and legumes are considered enhancement foods under the 28-MR. While they provide fiber, minerals, and other valuable nutrients, they are also relatively rich in carbohydrates. For this reason, they should complement the foundation of your plate rather than replace any of the main components.

Continue building meals around protein, vegetables, and healthy fats, and think of beans and legumes as supporting additions.

By now, you have experienced life with and without dairy. You have also had the opportunity to evaluate your response to beans and legumes. More importantly, you have spent nearly three weeks practicing a different way of eating and thinking about food. As you move into the final week of the 28-MR, the focus begins to shift from implementation to sustainability. The question is no longer whether you can complete this challenge. The question becomes how to carry what you have learned forward.

Week Four: Sustain and Transition

In the final days of the 28-MR approach, many participants begin to ask an important question: What happens next? After all, this program was never meant to just create a challenge. Instead, it was designed to build understanding, develop new skills, and invite participants to experience a different way of caring for themselves.

You have spent plenty of time using the Metabolic Restoration Filter, practicing Meal Architecture, prioritizing protein, reducing added sugar, avoiding gluten, improving hydration, and becoming more attuned to your body's feedback. You have also had the opportunity to evaluate your response to dairy, beans, and legumes. You have definitely gathered valuable new information.

The final week is not about introducing new rules. It is about deciding which habits, foods, and practices are worth keeping. Rather than asking, what can I start eating again? Consider asking a different question: What habits have improved my life enough that I no longer want to give them up?

For some people, the answer may be eating more protein. For others, it may be meal preparation, improved hydration, fewer processed foods, better sleep, or simply paying closer attention to how food affects their body. You might discover that you no longer want to return to habits you once had because you have experienced what it feels like to have your body consistently supported, and that new knowledge becomes a powerful guide for future decisions.

Measuring Your Progress

Before concluding the 28-MR, take a few minutes to complete the Post-Program Metabolic Assessment in Appendix B. One of the challenges with health improvement is that changes occur gradually. Common symptoms slowly become less noticeable, and improvements can be easily overlooked.

By comparing your responses from Appendix A and Appendix B, you will gain a clearer picture of the changes that occurred. The purpose of the assessment is not to achieve a perfect score. It is to help you recognize patterns, measure progress, and become more aware of your own wellness journey.

Health is not a Straight Line

Remember that health is rarely a straight line. Some people will complete the 28-MR and continue many of these habits for years to come. Others may gradually find themselves returning to some of their previous routines. Real life has a way of testing even the best intentions, and old habits can be exceptionally persistent. If that happens, do not make the mistake of believing that the 28-MR was unsuccessful.

Imagine two individuals. One completes the 28-MR and experiences four weeks of improved nutrition, hydration, and sleep, fewer processed foods, and greater insight into how their body responds to food. The other one decides not to begin because they are uncertain whether they can maintain the changes in the long term.

Even if the first person eventually drifts back toward old habits, they have still given their body something valuable. They have created a period of healing, recovery, and renewal that otherwise would not have existed. Just as importantly, they have gained knowledge through experience. They now know what is possible. They know how they felt when they consistently invest in their health, and they know they can return to those habits whenever they choose.

Rarely is a meaningful health transformation defined by a single effort. More often, it is shaped by many attempts, many lessons, and many opportunities to begin again. Every step toward better health matters, even when the path is not perfectly linear.

Whether this becomes the beginning of a lasting transformation or simply an important chapter in a longer process, your body will benefit enormously from the effort. Most importantly, you will leave with something no one can take away: the knowledge that positive change is possible.

You now have everything you need

At some point, preparation must give way to action. It is easy to tell yourself that you will start when life becomes less busy, when work settles down, when the holidays are over, or when someone decides to do it with you. The problem is that those conditions rarely occur.

Starting something new can feel uncomfortable. It may even feel a little intimidating. That is understandable. Most meaningful changes start that way. So, pick a date. Put it on your calendar and commit to it. Do not wait for perfect circumstances, more motivation, or for someone else to join you. Just begin.

Will the next four weeks be perfect? Probably not. Life rarely cooperates that way. There will always be reasons to postpone, interruptions to navigate, and excuses if you look for them. The only thing between where you are today and where you could be twenty-eight days from now is a decision. Make it. Twenty-eight days from now, you will be glad you did.

Getting Started with the 5-Day Gut Reset Program

If you would like a little extra guidance as you begin, I have created the **5-Day Gut Reset Program**, which walks you through the first five days of the Metabolic Restoration Program.

The Gut Reset follows the same nutritional principles presented in this book and corresponds to the opening days of the 28-day journey. Each day includes a short video where I explain the day's focus, answer common questions, and offer practical encouragement as you begin implementing these changes. While this program is completely optional, many readers find that having someone guide them through those first few days makes the transition feel simpler and more manageable. To access the 5-Day Gut Reset, simply scan the QR code below or visit:

https://l.bttr.to/RYjoV

Beyond the 28-MR

Long before I created the 28-Day Metabolic Restoration, I developed a program called the Juice Cleanse Reset (JCR). For over six years, and with hundreds of patients, I have used this vegetable juice and bone broth protocol with individuals seeking an intensive nutritional reset.

While the 28-MR is designed as a sustainable lifestyle framework, the JCR was created as a short-term intervention. The two programs share many of the same principles, including reducing reliance on ultra-processed foods, improving awareness of eating habits, and creating an opportunity to interrupt long-established patterns. However, they approach those outcomes in different ways.

The 28-MR focuses on building long-term habits and creating a way of eating that can realistically fit into everyday life. The JCR, on the other hand, is designed to temporarily simplify food choices and provide a period for a profound cleanse.

For some individuals, the 28-MR will be the ideal starting point. Others may choose to begin with the JCR and later transition into the 28-MR as a long-term lifestyle framework. I view these programs as complementary tools that can be used depending on an individual's preferences and health status. If you are interested in learning more, you will find the complete Juice Cleanse Reset protocol in Appendix E.

Chapter 11

A Different Vision for Health

★★★

The greatest medicine of all is to teach people how not to need it.
— Hippocrates

Prevention Is Not Sexy… Until It's Too Late

One of the greatest challenges with prevention is that it rarely feels urgent in the moment. Most people do not wake up thinking about preserving their health twenty years into the future. Daily responsibilities have a way of pushing health into the background until something demands attention and cannot be postponed any longer.

We tend to respond more strongly to a crisis than to slow, invisible change. A sudden diagnosis immediately reorganizes attention. Chest pain interrupts denial. Exhaustion that no longer improves forces people to pause in ways they may have avoided for years. Health, or the lack thereof, suddenly becomes real when the body can no longer be ignored, while prevention asks people to care long before consequences fully arrive.

The world around us reinforces this. Convenience, stimulation, speed, productivity, comfort, and instant gratification are rewarded everywhere. Caring for the future version of ourselves requires a very different mindset.

And yet, many of the habits that have the greatest influence on long-term health appear almost unimpressive in ordinary life. A walk rarely feels life-changing while it is happening. Neither does cooking at home, sleeping well consistently, preserving strength, or allowing space for meaningful recovery. Over time, ordinary daily choices, whether beneficial or detrimental, begin to shape the kind of future a person grows into.

When Health Stops Feeling Abstract

For most of history, simply living longer was considered a remarkable achievement. Advances in medicine, sanitation, emergency care, and technology have extended life expectancy in ways previous generations could hardly have imagined. Just one hundred years ago, life expectancy in the United States was around fifty-four years old[50]. People today routinely survive conditions that once ended lives much earlier. But as lifespan increased, a different question began emerging: What kind of life are those additional years creating?

The field of longevity medicine made an important distinction between surviving longer (lifespan) and remaining fully alive within those added years (healthspan). The conversation has shifted toward something deeper: preserving mobility, mental sharpness, purpose, connection, autonomy, and the ability to continue having a meaningful life.

As we grow older, health and decline stop feeling theoretical. For some, it begins with abnormal laboratory results or exhaustion that no longer improves with rest. For others, it arrives while watching a parent decline, receiving difficult news, or waking up one morning with the realization that the body no longer feels the same.

Those moments tend to reorganize priorities quickly. Sleep suddenly matters differently. Stress is no longer dismissed so casually. Time itself starts feeling more valuable. People begin paying attention not only to how long they may live, but to the kind of life they are building along the way.

One of the deepest shifts occurs when the question slowly changes from, "How do I look?" to, "How do I want to live for the rest of my life?" Very different choices begin unfolding from that place, usually alongside the quiet hope that change is not arriving too late.

Aging Is Not the Enemy

A damaging idea society has normalized is the belief that growing older is somehow a failure. Aging is often treated as something to resist, conceal, or delay. But aging itself is not the enemy. Growing older is a privilege many never receive. There is a meaningful difference between the natural passage of time and the decline that can follow decades of wear and neglect.

The visible signs of aging are part of being human. The body changes, and so do our priorities. Life leaves marks on all of us. But losing the ability to move comfortably through the world, withdrawing from experiences because the body no longer cooperates, or arriving in later years already exhausted and disconnected from daily life is not something people should automatically accept as inevitable. Over the years, the body reflects the conditions it has lived under through care or neglect repeated over a lifetime.

Longevity science is increasingly helping people understand that many aspects once assumed to be unavoidable parts of aging may be far more influenced by lifestyle and environment than previous generations believed. Not because we are meant to remain young forever, but because preserving physical and cognitive function allows people to remain active and independent participants of society for as long as possible. Moving comfortably, remaining mentally present, maintaining meaningful relationships, and staying curious about the world around us should remain part of the human experience for as long as possible, rather than becoming rare exceptions celebrated as good fortune.

Technology and the Human Body

Technology is transforming healthcare in ways that would have seemed unimaginable only a few decades ago. People can now monitor sleep, glucose, heart rhythms, recovery, movement, body composition, and a growing array of other biological metrics with remarkable precision. Artificial intelligence is beginning to assist clinicians in pattern recognition, while wearable devices allow individuals to observe in real time how their daily habits affect them.

And yet, despite access to more information than ever before, many feel increasingly out of touch with their own bodies. Information alone does not automatically create understanding. In some cases, constant tracking can even become another source of pressure, in which health shifts from a relationship with the body to a performance measured by numbers. A poor sleep score can shape the tone of the morning before the day even begins. A glucose spike may create guilt instead of curiosity. Recovery metrics can begin to influence mood more than they should, and, little by little, external data can overshadow internal awareness.

At the same time, these tools can become extraordinarily valuable when used with perspective. Many people have spent years functioning through chronic overstimulation and inflammation to the point that their internal baseline has quietly changed without them even realizing it.

Technology can help interrupt that adaptation. A person wears a continuous glucose monitor and begins to notice, in real time, how dramatically certain meals affect energy, concentration, and cravings throughout the day. Another begins consistently tracking sleep and can detect just how much inadequate rest had been affecting mood, recovery, focus, and resilience for years before it was ever consciously recognized. Changes that once remained invisible can now be observed directly and connected to daily choices with notable clarity.

Used thoughtfully, these tools can help individuals notice what their bodies have been trying to reveal for years, not by replacing intuition, but by helping them reconnect with it. They allow people to observe important signals earlier, better understand the effects of certain habits, and rebuild trust in their own internal awareness.

Fixing the Truck

Medicine continues to make extraordinary advances. In recent years, medications originally developed to help manage diabetes have transformed the conversation around weight loss and metabolic health.

GLP-1 medications have done something many never thought possible: they have quieted constant hunger, reduced cravings, and softened what many describe as "food noise[51]."

For some individuals, these medications can be life-changing. They may create enough physiological relief to finally allow healthier habits to take root. They can become valuable tools, particularly for people struggling with severe obesity, insulin resistance, or decades of metabolic dysfunction.

I am grateful that these options exist. At the same time, I believe these medications are most effective when they are part of a larger strategy rather than the entire strategy itself. Ideally, they should be prescribed thoughtfully by compassionate clinicians who understand nutrition, body composition, muscle preservation, metabolic health, and the realities of long-term behavior change.

The goal should never be simply to help someone eat less to lose weight. It should be to help them become healthier. For some individuals, these medications may become a long-term part of the plan. Others may be able to reduce or discontinue them as healthier alternatives become established. Every situation is different. What matters most is remembering that the medication is a tool, not the entire blueprint.

Not long ago, a patient shared a story with me about her diabetic father. She told me how happy he was after starting a GLP-1 medication because he could once again enjoy many of the foods he loved without seeing his blood sugar rise as dramatically. As she spoke, I found myself reflecting on the situation from a different perspective. As a clinician, I understand how meaningful that kind of relief can be. But I also found myself wondering whether we sometimes risk missing the larger opportunity. Healthcare should not be about developing enough medications to allow us to continue the behaviors that contributed to the problem in the first place.

That thought reminded me of something I witnessed one morning as I was leaving my neighborhood. I noticed a torn trash bag lying in the middle of the road. A few cars had already driven over it, and the contents were beginning to scatter across the street. This was obviously an isolated incident. Given enough time, traffic, wind, and rain would scatter the debris until little evidence remained.

But then I imagined something different. What if the same trash truck drove down that road every day and dropped a new bag daily? The city could continue sending cleanup crews. They could become remarkably efficient at removing the trash. They could hire more workers, purchase better equipment, and develop increasingly sophisticated ways of cleaning the street.

But eventually, someone would need to ask a different question. Why is the truck dropping the bags in the first place? Is there a hole in the truck? A mechanical failure? Something upstream that keeps creating the same problem over and over again?

In many ways, healthcare faces a similar challenge. We continue developing increasingly sophisticated ways to manage the consequences of metabolic dysfunction. Some of these advances are impressive and have improved both the quality and length of countless lives. But while treatment matters, prevention matters too. While cleanup crews are valuable, preventing the spill is often even better.

The future of medicine is not choosing between treatment and prevention. It is learning how to do both exceptionally well. We need the medications. We need the technology. We need innovation. But we also need to remain willing to ask why the truck keeps dropping the bags.

The Human Side of Prevention

A humbling aspect of preventive medicine is realizing that information alone is rarely enough to change behavior. For example, I have close friends who consistently make an effort to care for their health. And yet, despite all that awareness, they still find themselves pulled toward behaviors they do not fully understand.

One friend, despite being extraordinarily disciplined in many aspects of her nutrition, ate an entire Dubai chocolate bar intended for multiple servings three days in a row, even though she knew it would leave her physically unwell afterward. Another described feeling almost powerless around sugar despite years of reading about health, listening to podcasts, completing several juice fasts, and making major lifestyle changes. She spoke about it, nearly in tears, frustrated that understanding nutrition intellectually still did not quite address the intensity of the pull itself.

Stories like these inevitably raise difficult questions: Why do intelligent, self-aware people who sincerely want to change continue to engage in behaviors they consciously know are harming them? The answer is rarely straightforward.

Behavior is shaped by far more than knowledge alone. With repeated reinforcement, food can become deeply tied to comfort, relief, predictability, emotional regulation, or distraction. Years of self-soothing through food can leave imprints that information alone does not automatically erase. In some cases, addictive tendencies may also be involved. This is one reason shame rarely softens the struggle. What appears irrational on the surface is often connected to something much deeper.

There is another layer worth considering. Part of us may genuinely want change, while another part quietly resists it. We naturally gravitate toward what is familiar, even when it no longer serves us. Over time, behaviors, coping mechanisms, and ways of thinking can become so thoroughly woven into daily life that they begin to feel like part of who we are.

This is why change feels so uncomfortable. It is not a matter of learning something new. It often requires letting go of something deeply rooted. Lasting change begins when we acknowledge that a part of us may be holding on just as tightly as another part is trying to let go. Perhaps part of prevention is learning to approach these struggles not only with discipline, but also with enough honesty and compassion to ask deeper questions: "Why can't I stop?" "What am I truly trying to soothe, escape, replace, or quiet through this behavior?" and "What part of me is benefiting from keeping this pattern alive?"

A Blue Zone State of Mind

Having lived in several larger cities across the United States after growing up in Barcelona, I found that Las Cruces, New Mexico, was the smallest community I had ever lived in. After spending more than a decade here, I found certain commonalities in the way people lived, ate, moved, and cared for themselves increasingly difficult to ignore.

That perspective led me to reflect on communities commonly referred to as Blue Zones, places where everyday life naturally supports health through movement, nourishment, connection, purpose, sunlight, nature, and strong social relationships[52]. What fascinates me most about these communities is that healthy choices are not viewed as unusual. They are woven into the culture itself.

One evening, while talking with a close friend who is also deeply passionate about prevention, we found ourselves discussing this idea. We wondered how different people might feel physically and emotionally if healthier choices became part of their environment, rather than something individuals had to fight for on their own.

Las Cruces has a population of roughly 120,000 people[53]. Yet medical clinics, urgent care centers, pharmacies, and healthcare offices seem to be on nearly every corner, something my mother still finds striking whenever she visits from Spain. Despite the abundance of healthcare services, visible illness remains everywhere. Obesity, diabetes, cardiovascular disease, chronic pain, metabolic dysfunction, and physical decline have become so common that they no longer raise concern the way they should.

Sadly, many of the habits contributing to poor health have become an integral part of the landscape. Fast food surrounds schools. Sugary drinks become part of childhood. Highly processed meals become everyday convenience. Bringing donuts, candy, or junk food into workplaces is often associated with generosity, celebration, comfort, or simply being thoughtful toward others. Before long, the environment begins reinforcing the very behaviors that contribute to illness. But if unhealthy habits can spread through a community, perhaps healthy ones can as well.

Years ago, I witnessed a small version of this phenomenon unfold among a group of close friends. One of my dearest friends, Elisa, reached a point where she could not continue feeling the way she did. Like many women entering midlife, she was struggling with fatigue, poor sleep, aches and pains, weight gain, and the general feeling that her body no longer felt like her own.

For years, I had shared ideas about nutrition and health with my friends. I was usually the person bringing the healthier dish to a gathering or talking about ingredients while everyone else rolled their eyes and reached for soda and chips. They loved me, but most were not particularly interested in changing the way they ate.

Then one day, everything shifted. I was at Elisa's house having coffee when she told me she was done. She was tired of feeling tired. She had been praying for answers and had come across a Spanish doctor who taught a 21-day juice-fasting program (see Appendix E). She had decided she was going to do it.

I remember thinking there was no way she would make it all the way through. Not because she lacked determination, but because the change seemed so dramatic compared to the way she had eaten for most of her life.

A few days later, I called to check on her. Instead of sounding miserable, she sounded energized. She told me she was sleeping better. Her energy was improving. She had already lost weight. Most importantly, she sounded hopeful. I was shocked, but also pleasantly surprised.

Then something beautiful happened. The rest of our group of girlfriends started paying attention. Curiosity began to spread through the group, and several of us decided to try it ourselves. It's important to understand that these were not health fanatics. We were ordinary women with busy lives, imperfect eating habits, and a long history of enjoying bread, desserts, celebrations, comfort foods, and shared meals together.

Yet many of us completed the process. And it changed us — not only physically, but culturally. The conversations we had around food transformed, as did the recipes we shared. The meals we brought to gatherings changed. For a long time, discussions about health, wellness, and nutrition became a central part of our friendship.

Years later, many of those changes remain. Even one woman became interested in nutritional approaches to support her child's ADHD symptoms. What started as one woman making a decision for herself created a ripple effect that extended far beyond her own life.

I think about that experience often because it taught me something important. We tend to believe our choices affect only us. But health rarely works that way. One person's courage gives another person permission to try. One person's transformation creates curiosity. One person's example can influence an entire family, a group of friends, a workplace, or even a community. And this is how meaningful cultural change begins. It starts when ordinary people make different choices, and those choices become visible to those around them.

Because once enough individuals begin to change, the environment itself slowly changes too. Restaurants respond differently. Schools begin supporting health differently. Workplaces start offering healthier options. Conversations start to shift. Healthier living stops feeling unusual and starts feeling normal.

Children raised in that kind of environment would likely develop an entirely different relationship with food, movement, and self-care from the very beginning. Schools might emphasize nourishment more intentionally. Communities could invest more heavily in walking trails, parks, fitness studios, farmers' markets, cooking education, outdoor spaces, and wide access to wholesome food. That gives me enormous hope for the future of health.

Technology, artificial intelligence, personalized medicine, and longevity science will undoubtedly continue transforming healthcare in unprecedented ways. But some of the most meaningful progress may ultimately come from something far less technological and far more human: communities gradually changing what they normalize. Because true health is shaped far less inside hospitals than through the environments people live in every single day.

Chapter 12

The Spiritual Dimension of Health

✦✦✦

Until you make the unconscious conscious, it will direct your life, and you will call it fate.
— Carl Jung

Beyond the Body

Throughout this book, we have explored many of the factors that influence physical health. These subjects matter enormously because the body is the vehicle through which we experience every aspect of physical life.

When I first entered healthcare, I believed that if I learned enough science, physiology, pharmacology, and medicine, I would eventually understand most of what determines health. And to some degree, science does provide extraordinary answers. It explains how hormones influence mood, how inflammation contributes to disease, how sleep affects metabolism, and how lifestyle choices shape long-term outcomes.

Yet after years of caring for patients, I began noticing something that medicine alone could not fully explain. I met people whose laboratory results looked excellent on paper, yet they seemed disconnected from life itself. They moved through their days exhausted, discouraged, anxious, or searching for something they could not quite name. At the same time, I met people carrying significant health challenges who possessed a sense of peace, resilience, gratitude, and purpose that no laboratory value could measure.

Those observations forced me to ask questions that had little to do with diagnoses, prescriptions, or treatment plans. Why do some people maintain hope in circumstances that appear overwhelming, while others struggle despite having every apparent advantage? Why do some individuals transform their lives after a health scare, while others remain stuck even when they desperately want to change? Why can two people receive the same information and respond in completely different ways?

There is something about human experience that extends beyond what can be fully captured through science. At some point, nearly everyone begins asking questions that no data can answer. Why am I here? What does my life mean? What truly matters? What kind of person am I becoming?

Questions like these arise because being human involves more than surviving. We are not only biological beings trying to extend our lifespan. We are also searching for meaning, purpose, connection, and a sense that our lives matter.

The longer I practiced, the more difficult it became for me to separate physical health from the quality of a person's inner life. Somewhere along the way, my interest in health began leading me toward questions that science alone could not fully answer.

The Voice in Our Heads

One idea that fundamentally changed the way I understand both health and life began with a deceptively simple observation. Most of us spend our entire lives listening to a voice inside our heads. It comments on what is happening around us. It worries about the future. It replays conversations from the past. It criticizes, compares, judges, analyzes, plans, and narrates our experiences from the moment we wake up until the moment we fall asleep[54].

For many years, I assumed that voice was simply me. Then I encountered a question that stopped me in my tracks. If I can hear that voice, who is the one listening? At first, the question sounded strange. But the more I sat with it, the more fascinating it became.

Most of us have experienced moments when we suddenly become aware of our thoughts. In that moment, something interesting happens.

There is mental activity, and there is also that part of us that recognizes the thought. That realization suggests that we are not every thought that passes through our minds. When we learn to observe those mental patterns instead of automatically reacting to them, we create a small amount of space between stimulus and response. In that space, something important becomes possible: self-awareness. And that is where meaningful change begins.

Before someone changes their nutrition, they must first become aware of what they are eating. Before someone improves their sleep, they must acknowledge how tired they truly feel. Before someone transforms their health, they must notice the habits, assumptions, and recurring tendencies that shape their daily life. Self-awareness helps us see ourselves more clearly, making different choices possible.

Every idea explored throughout this book rests upon a simple but often overlooked truth: We cannot change what we do not notice. The first step is not action. The first step is recognition.

Your Body, Your Temple

Before continuing, I should acknowledge that what follows reflects my personal spiritual perspective. I recognize that readers may hold very different beliefs, and I respect that completely. My intention is not to persuade anyone to adopt my worldview, but to share some of the ideas that have shaped my understanding of health, healing, and life experience.

As my own spiritual perspective evolved over the years, certain teachings began resonating with me in ways they never had before. One of them was a simple statement attributed to Jesus: "The Kingdom of God is within you" (Luke 17:21). This short saying raises an extraordinary question. If the Kingdom of God is within us, what exactly does that mean? Is it simply symbolic language, or is it pointing toward something deeper about humans and our relationship with the divine? The more I contemplated those words, the more a different possibility emerged. What if the divine is not something distant, existing somewhere beyond us? What if there is something sacred already present within each one of us?

Another passage that captured my attention appears in the Gospel of John: "Is it not written in your law, 'I said, you are gods'?" (John 10:34). That statement raises an equally profound question. What did Jesus mean by those words? Was he speaking metaphorically, or was he inviting people to recognize a deeper truth about their own nature? I do not claim to have the answer. But I found the question impossible to ignore.

As I reflected on these ideas, I began seeing the body differently. No longer as a biological machine, a collection of organs, or a physical structure carrying us through life, but as something far more meaningful: a temporary home entrusted to our care.

When we think of a temple, we think of a place that holds significance. It is cared for because it matters. I began to see the body in the same light: something worthy of respect, attention, and gratitude.

Viewed through that lens, many of the ideas explored throughout this book begin to take on a different meaning. Food is no longer simply a source of pleasure, convenience, or fuel; it is one of the primary ways we care for and support ourselves. Movement offers an opportunity to strengthen and honor the physical vessel through which we experience life. Sleep provides a period of restoration, allowing the body and mind to recover and renew themselves. Caring for ourselves is no longer merely a health strategy. It becomes an expression of gratitude, responsibility, and respect for the life we have been given.

Whether one believes life comes from God, the universe, a higher intelligence, or a mystery beyond human understanding, the conclusion remains remarkably similar. This body is the only one entrusted to us for this chapter of our existence. It will change with the passing years, carry the stories of a life fully lived, and one day return to the earth. What remains within our control is how we choose to care for it while it is ours.

For me, that is one of the deepest reasons health matters. Caring for ourselves becomes a way of honoring God, expressing gratitude for the life we have been given, and making the most of the time we are granted in this physical form.

The Neighbor Within

Most people would never speak to a close friend the way they speak to themselves. If a friend made a mistake, we would usually respond with understanding. If someone we loved was struggling, we would offer encouragement rather than continually remind them of their weaknesses. Yet our internal dialogue is often far less forgiving. The voice directed inward can be relentless. It magnifies flaws, questions decisions, and demands standards we would rarely expect from anyone else.

One of the most widely known spiritual teachings from Jesus says: “Love your neighbor as yourself” (Matthew 22:39). What makes this so intriguing is the assumption hidden within it. Most discussions focus on “love your neighbor.” Far less attention is given to the rest of the phrase "as yourself." Yet those two words raise an important question: What if the way we relate to ourselves influences every other relationship in our lives? After all, the statement assumes that we know how to relate to ourselves in the first place. But what happens when we don't? What happens when the relationship closest to us is shaped by judgment, frustration, or a persistent sense of inadequacy? It becomes difficult to consistently offer others something largely absent from our own experience.

This is one reason self-care is so widely misunderstood. Many people confuse it with selfishness, when in reality the two have very little in common. Caring for our health, honoring our limits, allowing adequate rest, and treating ourselves with greater understanding do not diminish what we can offer the world. It expands it. A depleted person has less to give than a nourished one. Someone carrying resentment often struggles to extend patience. A person engaged in a constant internal battle may find it difficult to create harmony in relationships.

The way we relate to ourselves inevitably influences the way we move through the world. It shapes our conversations, our reactions, the assumptions we make about others, and the degree of generosity we bring into our daily interactions. Perhaps loving our neighbor begins much closer to home than we realize.

The Lesson Within the Struggle

Very few people welcome difficulty when it arrives. When life becomes painful, confusing, disappointing, or uncertain, the natural response is resistance. We want the problem solved, the discomfort removed, and the situation restored to its previous state. Yet many of the experiences that shape us most profoundly are not the ones we would have chosen.

Looking back on my own life, I can identify moments that felt very frustrating at the time but later revealed themselves to be important turning points. Relationships that ended. Plans that failed. Unexpected detours that pushed me in directions I never would have chosen voluntarily.

The same theme appears repeatedly throughout life. What initially feels like an obstacle sometimes becomes an opportunity for growth, even when it is disguised as disappointment, uncertainty, or loss.

What if life is not happening to us, but also teaching us? That question does not remove pain or make difficult circumstances easier. It does, however, invite a different perspective. Instead of asking only, "Why is this happening to me?" we begin asking, "What can I learn from this?"

The answer is rarely immediate. Sometimes understanding arrives much later. Occasionally, the meaning of an experience only becomes clear when viewed from a completely different chapter of life. Yet growth often emerges from circumstances that initially appear to offer nothing but struggle.

This does not mean that every setback exists to teach a lesson, nor that every challenge carries a hidden message waiting to be discovered. But periods of difficulty frequently reveal something important about us. They expose habits we were unaware of, assumptions we never questioned, fears we had avoided, or priorities that had drifted out of alignment. In that sense, adversity can become a powerful teacher. Not because suffering is inherently valuable, but because it reveals what comfort often conceals.

Health, too, can be part of that process. Sometimes the greatest transformations begin not when everything is going well, but when something forces us to pause, pay attention, and reconsider the way we are living. From that perspective, health becomes more than the absence of disease. It becomes part of a larger journey of learning, growth, and self-discovery.

My Life Purpose

Whether we are aware of it or not, each of us carries a purpose. We may not always see it clearly, and it may reveal itself gradually over the course of a lifetime, but it is there. Purpose is not reserved for a select few with extraordinary talents or obvious callings. It often expresses itself through the quiet ways we influence others, the choices we make, and the lives we touch along the way.

For a long time, I thought my purpose was to help people improve their health. Over the years, however, I have come to understand that health itself is not the final destination. Health is a vehicle. So is teaching nutrition, practicing medicine, and having conversations with patients every day.

What truly calls me is something deeper. I feel called to help people become more conscious—more aware of the choices they make each day, the patterns they repeat, and the future they are quietly building. Not everyone is ready for that awareness, and I have learned to respect that. Transformation cannot be forced. A person must arrive at that moment in their own time. But for those who are ready, I hope this work serves as an invitation. An invitation to wake up. To question what they have accepted as inevitable. To stop being carried by momentum.

I am not here to rescue or tell another person how to live, but rather to illuminate a path for those who are ready to see it. If this book helps even a few people become more conscious of the choices that shape their future, then it has fulfilled its purpose. And I will know that I am fulfilling mine.

Chapter 13

Full Circle

✦ ✦ ✦

Life can only be understood backward, but it must be lived forwards.
— Søren Kierkegaard

The Path I was Meant to Walk

If you had asked me twenty years ago whether I would someday write a book about health, wellness, and living well, I probably would have thought you were talking about someone else. At the time, writing a book was not part of my plans. Truthfully, healthcare was not part of my life either. My first degree was in International Business, and after graduation, I spent a few years working in that field. Later, I stepped away from my career to focus on raising my children. If someone had told me then where life was about to lead, I never would have believed them.

It all began with what seemed like a very ordinary experience. During a routine visit to an obstetrics and gynecology office, I encountered a staff member who made me feel unwelcome during an already vulnerable appointment. I remember leaving frustrated and telling my husband at the time how much a single interaction had affected my experience. "What does it take to do what she does?" I asked.

He explained that she was probably a medical assistant. I remember thinking that if one person could have that much impact on a patient, then perhaps I could too. My original plan was simple. I was going to become a medical assistant and show patients the kindness and respect I felt were missing from that encounter.

A few days later, a family friend who happened to be a Registered-Nurse suggested something different. "Why don't you become a nurse?" I knew almost nothing about nursing. But I said yes. That single conversation altered the course of my life. I began taking prerequisite classes and later enrolled in a vocational nursing program. I became a Licensed Vocational Nurse, then a Registered-Nurse, and later a Certified Nurse-Midwife. Somewhere along the way, I discovered that I loved learning about the body. What began as curiosity quickly became a passion.

I still remember studying physiology during those early years and feeling an excitement that is difficult to describe. There were moments when I would sit with a textbook and feel overwhelmed with gratitude for having found work that fascinated me so completely.

From there, the path unfolded in ways I never could have anticipated. I later became a Family Nurse Practitioner before completing my Doctor of Nursing Practice degree. What amazes me most is not the number of degrees. It is how much I loved the process. Every class, every clinical rotation, every new challenge expanded my understanding of what was possible.

Another turning point arrived years later when someone introduced me to a concept I knew almost nothing about: hormone replacement therapy. At first, I had little interest. Then I attended my first training. For three days, I sat at the edge of my seat. I could not believe what I was learning. I found myself asking the same question repeatedly: "How has nobody taught us this in school?"

That experience opened an entirely new world. Hormone optimization led me toward root-cause medicine and metabolic health. Metabolic health led me toward prevention, longevity, nutrition, sleep science, and the interconnected systems that influence human well-being. Each step built upon the one before it. In hindsight, I can see how every chapter of my journey contributed to the practitioner I eventually became.

As I cared for patients and taught these concepts for a long time, I found myself recommending books almost as often as I recommended supplements, laboratory tests, or lifestyle changes. Depending on the person sitting in front of me, I usually had a book I felt might help them continue learning long after our appointment ended. Occasionally, I would joke with myself that one day I should write my own. But it always felt like one of those ideas reserved for some distant future.

How This Book Found Me

This book arrived unexpectedly. It began during the first online 5-Day Gut Reset I led with a group of sixty-six participants. As the program unfolded, I found myself amazed by how eager people were to learn and how much valuable information had never been shared with them in a practical, understandable way. Important questions kept appearing in the chat. Conversations expanded in directions I had not anticipated. The more I taught, the more pieces started fitting together.

By the second day of the program, something unusual was happening. Initially, I started recording voice notes to myself with information that I thought might help improve future courses and educational materials. But the stream of thoughts did not stop. One voice note became ten. Ten became dozens. Before long, I had accumulated well over a hundred recordings containing observations, questions, insights, stories, and recurrent themes that seemed to be gathering into something I could not yet define.

It felt as though a door had opened. New insights were appearing faster than I could capture them. A conversation, a patient encounter, a question from a participant, or a quiet moment alone could suddenly trigger another train of thought. Some recordings contained only a sentence or two. Others unfolded into entire monologues. Topics that seemed unrelated would suddenly connect. Concepts I had taught for years began fitting together in ways I had never fully appreciated before.

At some point, I realized this was no longer course material. Something larger was taking shape. Three days after what felt like a whirlwind of inspiration, I sat down and began writing. What I expected to be a small project quickly became something much bigger.

For weeks, the book occupied a surprising amount of mental space. It was often the last thing I thought about before falling asleep and the first thing that greeted me when I woke up. Entire sections seemed to assemble themselves quietly in the background of my mind, waiting for an opportunity to be captured before they drifted away.

The experience felt unlike anything I had encountered before. Writing did not feel like another task to complete or another goal to accomplish. It felt more like participating in a conversation that had to take place. The paragraphs were not arriving fully formed, but the ideas, themes, and stories seemed to be organizing themselves beneath the surface. My job was to pay attention long enough to catch them.

Life continued as it always does. There was work to do, people to see, commitments to honor, and moments that deserved my full presence. Yet I continuously felt a steady pull back toward the manuscript waiting on my computer. Not because I was trying to finish it as quickly as possible, but because the process itself felt deeply meaningful.

A Grateful Heart

As I sit here writing these final pages, the emotion I feel most strongly is not pride. It is gratitude. Gratitude for a path I never could have planned. Above all, gratitude for having found work that I genuinely love.

Sometimes it still amazes me that a single doctor's appointment could eventually lead me here. At the time, I had no way of knowing that one uncomfortable experience would alter the direction of my life. I took the next step that felt right, and then the next. Years later, those small steps became a profession, a calling, and ultimately a life that has brought me immense fulfillment.

Writing this book has reminded me of the same curiosity that first drew me into healthcare. The desire to understand how the body works, to keep learning, and to help people feel better. That curiosity has never really left me. If anything, it has grown stronger with time.

Finishing this book feels less like the completion of a project and more like the beginning of a new chapter that is still unfolding. That is one of the things I appreciate most about this field: no matter how much we learn, there is always another layer waiting to be explored.

Looking back, I would not change any of it. Not the long nights studying nor the years spent in school. Not the sacrifices that were required along the way, and not even the unexpected detours that seemed inconvenient at the time.

Each experience contributed to something valuable. Each step prepared me for the next one. And somehow, all of those steps eventually led here. To these pages and this moment. And to the honor of knowing that you are reading these words. For that, I am deeply grateful.

A Final Word

Before you close this book, there is one final thing I would like to say. I do not know where you are on your journey right now. Perhaps you picked up this book because you were frustrated with the way you felt. Perhaps you were searching for answers, trying to understand your body, or looking for a different perspective on health. Maybe I or someone else recommended these pages to you. However they found their way into your hands, I am glad our paths crossed.

If there is one thing I hope you take away, it is not a specific diet, supplement, laboratory test, or protocol. Those things can be useful, and many of them have the potential to improve your health in meaningful ways. But the deeper message is much simpler. Your body is not fighting you; it is fighting FOR you.

For years, I have met people who felt betrayed by their bodies. They felt frustrated by symptoms, discouraged by weight gain, confused by changing hormones, or convinced that their best years were already behind them. Yet time and again, I have witnessed the remarkable ability of the body to respond when given the support it needs.

I hope that, even in a small way, my words have encouraged you to become more curious about your health, more engaged in your own well-being, and more confident in your ability to influence the direction of your future. You do not need to have all the answers; you just need to begin where you are.

If I have inspired even one positive change in your life, then every hour spent writing this work was worthwhile. My wish for you is simple: that you continue asking questions, continue learning, and continue caring for yourself with the same kindness and attention you would offer someone you deeply love.

And wherever life leads you next, I wish you health, purpose, and the courage to keep growing.

With love,
Vanessa Menanteau

Continue Your Metabolic Restoration Journey

Join the free Metabolic Restoration Community! The journey doesn't end with the last page of this book.

Scan the QR code to join the **Metabolic Restoration Community** and receive practical resources to help you continue building your health.

As a member, you'll receive:

✓ Early access to exclusive events & updates about new books
✓ New metabolism-supportive recipes
✓ Practical nutrition and longevity tips
✓ Occasional encouragement and inspiration to help you stay on track

I value your inbox. You'll hear from me about once a month, and only when I have something genuinely helpful to share.

If this book has made a difference in your life, I'd love to hear from you. Feel free to share your experience, your progress, or any insights you've gained along the way: MetabolicRestoration@EternaDoc.com.

If you're comfortable with it, please let me know if I may share your story or comments anonymously in future books, newsletters, or educational materials to inspire others on their own health journeys. While I may not be able to respond personally to every email, please know that your message is deeply appreciated.

I look forward to continuing this journey with you.
— Dr. Vanessa Menanteau

Looking for Personalized Guidance?

While this book is designed to help you better understand and improve your metabolic health, every individual has a unique story. In some cases, a personalized review can help identify the factors contributing to persistent symptoms and clarify the next steps.

If you'd like an individualized assessment, I offer **Metabolic Restoration Consultations** designed to complement—not replace—the care you receive from your healthcare team. My goal is to help you better understand your health, provide evidence-based, personalized recommendations, and develop a roadmap you can implement in collaboration with your primary care provider or specialist.

A consultation may include:

- A comprehensive review of your medical history and current concerns
- Personalized laboratory recommendations and orders
- An in-depth interpretation of your results
- Nutrition, lifestyle, and metabolic recommendations tailored to your needs
- A written action plan to help guide discussions with your healthcare provider

To learn more, visit:

www.EternaDoc.com

Appendix A

Metabolic Restoration Symptom Assessment (Pre-Program)

Today's date: ___________

Rate each symptom from 0 to 3
(0 = Never, 1 = Mild/occasional, 2 = Moderate, 3 = Severe)

Signs and Symptoms	0	1	2	3
Fatigue/loss of energy				
Loss of well-being or motivation				
Mood swings				
Anxiety				
Depressed mood				
Headaches				
Brain fog				
Memory problems				
Insomnia				
Sugar cravings				
Afternoon energy crashes				
Difficulty losing weight				
Weight gain				
Feeling cold all the time				
Bloating				
Constipation				
Acid reflux/GERD				
Painful joints				
Painful muscles				
Frequent infections or illnesses				
Acne				
Sexual dysfunction/Low libido				
Infertility				
Total Score For each Column:				
Total Score from this page:				

APPENDIX A

Women Only:				
Signs and Symptoms	**0**	**1**	**2**	**3**
Abnormal Vaginal bleeding				
Breast tenderness				
Pre-menstrual symptoms				
Frequent yeast infections				
Hot flashes				
Night sweats				
Total Score For each Column:				
Total Score from this page:				

Pre-Program Total:

Appendix B

Metabolic Restoration Symptom Assessment (Post-Program)

Today's date: ____________

Rate each symptom from 0 to 3
(0 = Never, 1 = Mild/occasional, 2 = Moderate, 3 = Severe)

Signs and Symptoms	0	1	2	3
Fatigue/loss of energy				
Loss of well-being or motivation				
Mood swings				
Anxiety				
Depressed mood				
Headaches				
Brain Fog				
Memory problems				
Insomnia				
Sugar cravings				
Afternoon energy crashes				
Difficulty losing weight				
Weight gain				
Feeling cold all the time				
Bloating				
Constipation				
Acid reflux/GERD				
Painful joints				
Painful muscles				
Frequent infections or illnesses				
Acne				
Sexual dysfunction/Low libido				
Infertility				
Total Score For each Column:				
Total Score from this page:				

Women Only:				
Signs and Symptoms	0	1	2	3
Abnormal Vaginal bleeding				
Breast tenderness				
Pre-menstrual symptoms				
Frequent yeast infections				
Hot flashes				
Night sweats				
Total Score For each Column:				
Total Score from this page:				

Post-Program Total:

Pre-Program Total:

Difference:

Compare Your Results

Congratulations on completing the 28-Day Metabolic Restoration Program. Now compare your **Pre-Program Total** from Appendix A with your **Post-Program Total** from Appendix B.

Many participants notice meaningful improvements in symptoms such as energy, sleep, mood, cravings, digestion, weight management, and overall well-being after completing the program.

Remember that progress is not always reflected by a single symptom. Small improvements across multiple areas can add up to a significant improvement in how you feel and function every day. Take a moment to celebrate your progress and reflect on how far you've come throughout this journey. Every positive change is a step toward better health, greater vitality, and a stronger foundation for long-term wellness.

Appendix C

Metabolic Restoration Recipes

The recipes in this section are not meant to turn you into a chef. They're simply practical examples of how the concepts from this book can look on a plate.

For many people, changing the way they eat isn't about learning what to do; it's about knowing what to make instead. If breakfast has always meant cereal, bagels, pastries, oatmeal, or a quick stop at the drive-through, it can be difficult to picture a different option. That's why you'll find several breakfast ideas designed to help you start your day with more protein.

The lunch and light meal section offers simple options for busy days, but don't overlook one of the easiest strategies of all: leftovers. Many of the dinner recipes work beautifully as next-day lunches, saving both time and effort.

As you explore the dinner recipes, you'll notice a common theme. They are built around a quality protein, accompanied by vegetables and naturally occurring healthy fats—the same Meal Architecture we've discussed in Chapter 10. Feel free to make these recipes your own. Swap vegetables, experiment with different proteins, adjust seasonings, and adapt them to your preferences and lifestyle. Become comfortable creating simple, nourishing meals that work for you.

You'll also notice that many of these recipes use an air fryer. Over the years, it has become one of my favorite kitchen tools because it's fast, easy to clean, and produces consistently delicious results. If you don't own an air fryer, don't worry; nearly every recipe can be adapted for the oven or stovetop with only minor adjustments. Use whichever method fits your kitchen and your lifestyle.

As your confidence grows, I encourage you to continue exploring recipes beyond this book. Searching for terms such as "low-carb," "keto," or "high-protein" can be a helpful starting point. Most importantly, continue applying the same filters you've learned throughout the 28-Day Metabolic Restoration Program. Over time, you'll find that choosing meals becomes less confusing and more intuitive.

Breakfast

HEARTY BREAKFAST PLATE

If you're not sure what to eat for breakfast, start here. Simple ingredients, minimal preparation, and plenty of flexibility make it an easy option for busy mornings. It's proof that a complete breakfast doesn't have to be complicated. Makes 1 serving.

Ingredients:
- 2-3 large eggs
- 1 teaspoon extra-virgin olive oil
- 1 cup mushrooms, sliced
- 2 cups fresh spinach
- ½ avocado, sliced
- ½ cup cherry tomatoes, halved (or 1 medium tomato, diced)
- Sea salt and black pepper to taste

Instructions:
1. Heat the olive oil in a skillet over medium heat.
2. Add the mushrooms and cook for 4–5 minutes, until softened and lightly browned.
3. Add the spinach and cook for 1–2 minutes, until wilted.
4. Season the vegetables with a pinch of sea salt and black pepper.
5. Prepare the eggs however you prefer: scrambled, over easy, sunny-side up, or as an omelet.
6. Transfer the mushrooms, spinach, and eggs to a plate.
7. Add the avocado and tomatoes on the side.
8. Season the tomatoes with a pinch of sea salt and a drizzle of extra-virgin olive oil.
9. Serve immediately and enjoy.

★ Dr. V's special tip:
This is more of a template than a recipe. Don't have mushrooms? Use zucchini. Don't have spinach? Try arugula, kale, or another leafy green. The goal is simply to include protein, vegetables, and healthy fats on your plate.

One habit that has made the biggest difference for me is to stop thinking about breakfast foods and start thinking about balanced meals. Eggs and vegetables make a wonderful breakfast, but they also make a wonderful lunch or dinner.

APPENDIX C

POWERHOUSE MORNING BOWL

This is my favorite breakfast and one I find myself returning to again and again. Packed with protein, fiber, healthy fats, and nutrient-dense ingredients, it keeps me satisfied for hours while providing an energizing start to the day. I know some of these ingredients may not already be sitting in your pantry, but think of this bowl as an investment in your health. Many of these staples can be used in other recipes, and once you have them on hand, putting this breakfast together takes just a few minutes. Makes 1 serving.

Ingredients:

- ⅓ cup plain kefir (about 80 grams)
- ½ cup frozen blueberries
- 1 scoop whey protein concentrate (about 20–25 grams protein)
- 1 scoop collagen peptides
- 2 tablespoons chia seeds
- 1 tablespoon hemp seeds
- 1 tablespoon walnuts, chopped
- 2 teaspoons unsweetened shredded coconut
- 1 teaspoon sesame seeds
- ½ teaspoon ground cinnamon
- 8 drops pure liquid stevia

Instructions:

1. Add the kefir, whey protein, collagen peptides, chia seeds, hemp seeds, walnuts, shredded coconut, sesame seeds, cinnamon, and stevia to a bowl.
2. Whisk until well combined.
3. Mix in the blueberries and let the bowl sit for about 15 minutes to allow the chia seeds to expand and the berries to thaw.

<u>★ Dr. V's special tip:</u>

Don't let the ingredient list intimidate you. Start with the basics and add ingredients as your pantry grows. If you don't have kefir, plain full-fat Greek yogurt works beautifully. You may want to thin it with a splash of milk to achieve a similar consistency.

If you'd like to take things one step further, consider making your own kefir at home. That's what I do. Homemade kefir is surprisingly simple to make, can be more economical than store-bought, and may contain a wider variety of beneficial bacteria and yeasts than some commercial versions. All you need are kefir grains and milk. Kefir grains can be found online, including through retailers such as Amazon, or sometimes through local health-conscious communities where people share extra grains. If making your own kefir feels overwhelming, don't worry; store-bought plain kefir is still an excellent choice.

During the dairy-free week of the 28-Day Metabolic Restoration Plan, simply replace the kefir or Greek yogurt with plain coconut yogurt.

APPENDIX C

MORNING RUSH SMOOTHIE

Some mornings call for a sit-down breakfast. Others don't. This smoothie is my answer for busy mornings when I need something quick and satisfying. Made from simple ingredients, it delivers approximately 50 grams of protein per serving without relying on a premade shake. Makes 1 serving.

Ingredients:

- 1 cup unsweetened cashew milk (or other unsweetened milk)
- ⅓ cup whey protein concentrate (28 grams)
- 1 serving unflavored collagen peptides (20 grams; about 4 tablespoons)
- ½ banana
- 2 tablespoons natural peanut butter or almond butter
- 1 tablespoon chia seeds
- 1 tablespoon unsweetened shredded coconut
- ½ teaspoon ground cinnamon
- 8 drops liquid stevia (optional)
- 1 cup ice

Instructions:

1. Add all ingredients to a blender.
2. Blend until smooth and creamy.
3. Pour into a glass and enjoy immediately.

✯ Dr. V's special tip:

If you're not hungry first thing in the morning, pour the smoothie into an insulated tumbler and take it with you. A good insulated container will keep it cold for hours, allowing you to sip it throughout the morning.
When purchasing peanut butter or almond butter, look for products with the simplest possible ingredient list. Ideally, the only ingredients should be peanuts or almonds, with perhaps a little salt. Avoid products with added sugars, vegetable oils, or unnecessary additives.

APPENDIX C

VEGGIE & BACON EGG BITES

These are a wonderful make-ahead breakfast idea. Keep a batch in the refrigerator, and you'll always have something ready for busy mornings. They're easy to customize and reheat beautifully throughout the week. Makes 12 egg bites.

Ingredients:

- 10 large eggs
- ½ cup cottage cheese
- 4 slices crispy bacon, chopped
- 1 cup mushrooms, finely chopped
- ½ yellow bell pepper, finely chopped
- 3 green onions (scallions), thinly sliced
- ½ teaspoon sea salt
- ¼ teaspoon black pepper
- ½ teaspoon chili powder
- ½ teaspoon of baking power
- Extra-virgin olive oil or avocado oil for greasing the muffin pan

Instructions:

1. Preheat the oven to 350°F.
2. Lightly grease a 12-cup muffin pan.
3. In a bowl, combine the mushrooms, bell peppers, green onions, salt, black pepper, and chili powder.
4. Divide the vegetable mixture evenly among the muffin cups.
5. Sprinkle the chopped bacon over the vegetables.
6. In a large bowl, whisk together the eggs, cottage cheese, and baking powder until well combined.
7. Pour the egg mixture evenly into the muffin cups, filling each about ¾ full.
8. Bake for 20–25 minutes, or until the eggs are set and lightly golden on top.
9. Allow to cool for a few minutes before removing from the muffin tin.

10. Serve warm or store in the refrigerator in an airtight container for up to 4 days.

★ Dr. V's special tip:

My favorite way to cook bacon is in the air fryer. Simply place a parchment paper liner designed for your air fryer basket in the bottom of the tray, arrange the bacon in a single layer, and cook at 400°F for 8–10 minutes, or until crisp. The parchment paper catches the grease, making cleanup incredibly easy.

One of the best things about egg bites is how versatile they are. Feel free to swap the vegetables based on what you have available. Spinach, zucchini, broccoli, or leftover roasted vegetables all work beautifully.

I often make a batch at the beginning of the week and keep it in the refrigerator for a quick breakfast. To reheat, place the egg bites in the air fryer at 400°F for about 8–10 minutes. They develop a lightly crisp exterior while staying tender inside and are often even better the next day.

APPENDIX C

APPLE & BERRY PROTEIN PANCAKES

If I'm going to eat pancakes, they need to earn their place on the plate. These pancakes are packed with protein, fiber, and wholesome ingredients, making them far more satisfying than traditional pancakes. Sweet blueberries, crisp apples, crunchy pecans, and warm cinnamon create layers of flavor and texture, while the warm berry sauce provides a delicious alternative to syrup. Best of all, this recipe contains no added sugar and gets its sweetness from fruit and allulose. Makes 8 pancakes.

Ingredients:

For the pancakes:

- 1 cup old-fashioned rolled oats
- 1 cup cottage cheese
- 3 large eggs
- 1 scoop whey protein concentrate (⅓ cup)
- 2 tablespoons chia seeds
- 1 teaspoon baking powder
- 1 tablespoon allulose
- 2 teaspoons ground cinnamon
- ¼ teaspoon sea salt
- ⅛ teaspoon ground nutmeg
- 1 medium Fuji apple, grated or finely diced
- 1 cup blueberries
- ½ cup pecans, chopped
- Butter to grease the pan

For the warm berry sauce:

- 1 cup frozen mixed berries
- 1 tablespoon water
- 1 tablespoon allulose

Instructions:

1. Add the oats, cottage cheese, eggs, whey protein, chia seeds, baking powder, allulose, cinnamon, salt, and nutmeg to a blender.

2. Blend until smooth.
3. Transfer the batter to a bowl and fold in the grated or finely diced apple, blueberries, and chopped pecans.
4. Let the batter rest for 5 minutes.
5. Meanwhile, prepare the berry sauce. Add the frozen berries, water, and allulose to a small saucepan.
6. Cook over medium-low heat for 10 minutes, stirring occasionally, until the berries soften and begin to break down.
7. Carefully transfer the berry mixture to a blender and blend until smooth. Serve warm.
8. Heat a skillet over medium heat and add a small amount of butter. As the pancakes cook, add more butter as needed between batches.
9. Pour about ½ cup batter per pancake onto the skillet.
10. Cook for 2–3 minutes, until bubbles begin to form and the edges start to set.
11. Flip and cook for an additional 2–3 minutes, until golden-brown and cooked through.
12. Serve warm, topped with the berry sauce.

★ Dr. V's special tip:

These pancakes freeze beautifully. Allow them to cool completely, then store them in an airtight container or freezer bag. When you're ready to enjoy them, simply thaw them and warm them in a toaster, toaster oven, or air fryer.

Light Fare

NOURISHING SALAD BOWL

This is one of the simplest and most versatile meals I make for myself. It comes together in minutes and provides a beautiful combination of fresh vegetables, healthy fats, protein, fiber, and fermented foods. The ingredients can be adjusted based on what you have available, making this recipe easy to enjoy year-round.

Ingredients:

- 2 cups mixed greens (such as arugula, spring mix, or baby greens)
- ½ cup shredded carrots
- ½ cup cherry tomatoes, halved
- 2 tablespoons sauerkraut or fermented vegetables
- 2 organic hard-boiled eggs, chopped
- ½ avocado, diced
- 1 tablespoon pumpkin seeds
- 2 teaspoons sesame seeds
- 1 tablespoon extra-virgin olive oil
- 2 teaspoons balsamic glaze
- Sea salt and black pepper to taste

Instructions:

1. Add the mixed greens to a large bowl.
2. Top with the shredded carrots, cherry tomatoes, sauerkraut, avocado, pumpkin seeds, and sesame seeds.
3. Add the chopped hard-boiled eggs.
4. Drizzle with the olive oil and balsamic glaze.
5. Season with sea salt and black pepper, if desired.
6. Enjoy as assembled!

APPENDIX C

★Dr. V's special tip:

I often use a simpler version of this salad to add more vegetables to my meals. Before lunch or dinner, I'll make a small bowl with mixed greens, shredded carrots, sauerkraut, pumpkin seeds, extra-virgin olive oil, and a drizzle of balsamic glaze. It's an easy habit that helps me increase my vegetable intake without much effort.

How I Make Hard-Boiled Eggs:

Hard-boiled eggs are one of my favorite foods to keep on hand. They're portable, inexpensive, rich in protein, and make an easy addition to salads, snacks, or quick meals.

1. Place 5 eggs in a saucepan in a single layer.
2. Cover the eggs with warm water.
3. Bring the water to a boil.
4. Once the water reaches a boil, set a timer for 15 minutes.
5. Drain the hot water and immediately cover the eggs with very cold water. For faster cooling, add a handful of ice cubes.
6. Once cooled, store the eggs in the refrigerator for up to one week.

My favorite peeling trick:

If you've ever struggled to peel a hard-boiled egg, gently tap it on the counter until small cracks cover most of the shell. Then slide the edge of a spoon between the shell and the egg and work your way around the surface. The shell often comes off in large pieces, making peeling much faster and less frustrating.

APPENDIX C

CURRIED BUTTERNUT SQUASH SOUP

This creamy soup is a delicious way to enjoy butternut squash. Roasting it first brings out its natural sweetness, while warming spices like curry, ginger, and cinnamon create a rich depth of flavor. The result is a comforting soup that's rich, flavorful, and perfect for cooler days. This is an easy recipe to prepare ahead of time and enjoy throughout the week. Makes 4 servings.

Ingredients:

- 1 medium butternut squash
- 1 tablespoon ghee
- 1 medium onion, finely chopped
- 2 medium carrots, finely chopped
- 1 tablespoon curry powder
- 1 teaspoon ground ginger
- 1 teaspoon sea salt
- ¼ teaspoon black pepper
- Pinch of cayenne pepper
- Pinch of ground cinnamon
- 3 cups chicken bone broth
- 1 cup canned full-fat coconut milk

Instructions:

1. Wrap the butternut squash in aluminum foil and place it in the air fryer at 375°F for about 40 minutes, or until tender. Allow it to cool enough to handle.
2. Remove the foil, cut the squash in half, scoop out the seeds, and remove the skin. Set the roasted squash aside.
3. In a large pot, melt the ghee over medium heat.
4. Add the curry powder, ginger, salt, black pepper, cayenne pepper, and cinnamon. Stir for about 60 seconds, until fragrant.
5. Add the onion. Cook for 5–7 minutes, stirring occasionally, until softened.
6. Add the carrots, roasted squash, and bone broth. Bring to a boil, then let it simmer gently for 20 minutes.

7. Carefully transfer the soup to a blender and blend until completely smooth.
8. Return the soup to low heat and stir in the coconut milk.
9. Heat gently for a few minutes. Serve warm, topped with a sprinkle of pumpkin seeds.

★ Dr. V's special tip:

Ghee is simply clarified butter, meaning the milk solids have been removed. It has a rich, buttery flavor and a higher smoke point than butter, making it excellent for cooking. If you don't have ghee, you can substitute extra-virgin olive oil.

Because I like my meals to include a source of protein, I often pair this soup with a couple of hard-boiled eggs or another simple protein source.

APPENDIX C

90-SECOND ALMOND FLOUR BREAD WITH SARDINES

Sometimes you simply want bread. This quick almond flour bread comes together in just a few minutes and can be used as a base for countless simple meals. Paired with tomatoes, olive oil, and sardines, it becomes a satisfying light meal packed with protein and Mediterranean flavor. Best of all, there is no kneading, rising, or baking required. Makes 1 serving.

Ingredients:

For the bread:

• 1 tablespoon extra-virgin olive oil
• 3 tablespoons almond flour
• ½ teaspoon baking powder
• 1 teaspoon sesame seeds
• Pinch of sea salt
• Pinch of dried rosemary
• 1 large egg

For serving:

• 1 medium tomato, sliced
• Extra-virgin olive oil for drizzling
• Sea salt to taste
• 1 can sardines packed in olive oil

Instructions:

1. In a small 1-cup microwave-safe glass container, combine the olive oil, almond flour, baking powder, sesame seeds, salt, rosemary, and egg.
2. Whisk until a smooth batter forms. A fork works well if you don't have a whisk.
3. Microwave for 90 seconds.
4. Carefully remove the container from the microwave and allow it to cool for a minute or two.
5. Gently remove the bread from the container and transfer it to a cooling rack or plate.
6. Once cool enough to handle, slice the bread in half.

7. Top each half with sliced tomato.
8. Drizzle generously with extra-virgin olive oil and sprinkle with sea salt.
9. Serve alongside the sardines or place the sardines directly on top of the bread.

★ Dr. V's special tip:

Think of this recipe as a foundation rather than a fixed meal. If sardines aren't your thing, try topping the bread with tuna, hard-boiled eggs, cottage cheese, cream cheese, avocado, or your favorite protein. The bread itself is incredibly versatile and can be used anywhere you might normally reach for toast, crackers, or sandwich bread. The bread can also be toasted in a toaster oven or air fryer for a few minutes after slicing if you prefer a firmer texture.

APPENDIX C

SPANISH-INSPIRED TUNA SALAD

This is one of the simplest meals I grew up eating in Spain. When tomatoes are ripe and flavorful, very little else is needed. The combination of tomatoes, tuna, cucumber, hard-boiled eggs, and a simple olive oil dressing creates a light, satisfying meal that comes together in just minutes. Makes 2 servings.

Ingredients:

- 2 cups mixed-color cherry or grape tomatoes, halved
- ½ cucumber, peeled, seeded, and sliced
- ¼ medium red onion, thinly sliced
- 2 hard-boiled eggs, sliced
- 10 ounces can of tuna packed in olive oil, drained
- 1 tablespoon extra-virgin olive oil
- 1 teaspoon balsamic vinegar or balsamic glaze
- Sea salt and black pepper to taste
- 1 teaspoon sesame seeds
- 2 tablespoons fresh parsley, finely chopped

Instructions:

1. Place the tomatoes, cucumber slices, and red onion in a bowl.
2. Drizzle with olive oil and balsamic vinegar or balsamic glaze.
3. Season with sea salt and black pepper and toss gently.
4. Top with the sliced hard-boiled eggs and tuna.
5. Sprinkle with sesame seeds and fresh parsley.

✯ Dr. V's special tip:

The quality of the tomatoes and tuna makes all the difference in this recipe. Whenever possible, choose ripe, in-season tomatoes and tuna packed in olive oil. Albacore tuna is delicious, but the best choice is often simply the highest-quality tuna available to you.

This salad can easily be prepared ahead of time and stored in the refrigerator. It's also a wonderful recipe to double for meal prep, making tomorrow's lunch just as easy as today's.

Dinner Favorites

BETTER BURGER DINNER

Who says a hamburger has to come in a bun? At its core, a hamburger is simply a seasoned beef patty. In this version, the burger takes center stage, accompanied by crispy homemade fries and a generous serving of broccoli. The result is a wholesome meal that delivers all the enjoyment of burger night while keeping the focus on the foods that nourish us most. Makes 2 servings.

Ingredients:

For the burgers:

- ½ pound organic ground beef
- 1 teaspoon Dr. V's Paprika Seasoning (see last recipe in this section)

For the fries:

- 2 medium potatoes, cut into fries
- 1 tablespoon extra-virgin olive oil
- Sea salt to taste

For the broccoli:

- 1 large head of broccoli, cut into florets
- Extra-virgin olive oil for serving
- Sea salt to taste

Instructions:

1. Preheat the air fryer to 350°F.
2. Wash potatoes well, without peeling them, and cut into a French fry shape. Place the potatoes in a bowl. Drizzle with olive oil, season with salt, and toss to coat.

3. Line the air fryer basket with parchment paper if desired. Arrange the fries in a single layer and cook for 20–25 minutes, stirring once halfway through, until golden and crisp. Set aside.
4. Increase the air fryer temperature to 400°F.
5. In a bowl, combine the ground beef with Dr. V's Paprika Seasoning. (If you haven't prepared the seasoning yet, use the individual spices listed above.)
6. Mix gently and form into two patties.
7. Place the patties on parchment paper and lightly drizzle them with extra-virgin olive oil, then place them in the air fryer and cook for approximately 10 minutes, or until they reach your preferred level of doneness.
8. While the burgers cook, bring water to a boil in a pot. Add the broccoli florets and cook until tender-crisp, about 4–5 minutes. Drain well.
9. If needed, return the fries to the air fryer for 1–2 minutes to rewarm.
10. Divide the burgers, fries, and broccoli between two plates. Drizzle the broccoli with extra-virgin olive oil and season with a pinch of sea salt before serving.

★Dr. V's special tip:

Pre-cut parchment paper liners designed to fit the shape of your air fryer can make cleanup incredibly easy. And don't be afraid to make this meal your own. Feel free to top your burger with cheese, sautéed mushrooms, bacon, or your favorite toppings. The beauty of a meal like this is its flexibility. The protein, vegetables, and healthy fats remain the foundation, while the details can be adapted to your taste.

APPENDIX C

STUFFED BELL PEPPERS & GREEN BEANS

These stuffed bell peppers are one of those meals that look impressive but require very little hands-on work. Sweet roasted bell peppers are filled with a simple savory beef mixture, topped with melted cheese, and paired with tender green beans for a colorful, wholesome meal. Best of all, this recipe makes excellent leftovers, making tomorrow's lunch or dinner just as delicious as today's. Makes 2 generous servings or 4 smaller servings.

Ingredients:

For the stuffed peppers:

- ½ pound ground beef
- 2 large orange bell peppers
- 3 green onions (scallions), sliced
- 1 tablespoon extra-virgin olive oil
- 1 teaspoon sea salt
- ½ teaspoon black pepper
- 1 cup shredded cheese of choice (cheddar, Monterey Jack, mozzarella, or Parmesan)

For the green beans:

- 1 pound fresh green beans, trimmed and washed
- Extra-virgin olive oil for serving
- Sea salt to taste

Instructions:

Prepare the beef filling:

1. Heat the olive oil in a large skillet over medium heat.
2. Add the sliced green onions, sauté for 5 minutes, until softened.
3. Add the ground beef. Using a spatula, break the meat into small crumbles as it cooks.
4. Season with salt and pepper.
5. Cook until the beef is fully browned and cooked through, about 8–10 minutes.

6. Remove from heat.

Prepare the peppers:

1. Wash the bell peppers thoroughly.
2. Cut each pepper in half lengthwise.
3. Remove the stem, seeds, and membranes from each half.
4. Divide the beef mixture evenly among the four pepper halves, pressing gently to fill them.

Air fry:

1. Preheat the air fryer to 350°F.
2. Arrange the stuffed pepper halves in the air fryer basket.
3. Cook for 30-35 minutes, or until bell peppers are tender.
4. Open the air fryer and sprinkle the cheese over each pepper.
5. Continue cooking the peppers in the air fryer for an additional 5 minutes, or until the cheese is melted and lightly golden.

Prepare the green beans:

1. While the peppers are cooking, bring a pot of water to a boil.
2. Add the green beans and cook for 8-10 minutes, or until tender.
3. Drain well.
4. Drizzle with extra-virgin olive oil and season with sea salt.

Serve: Place two stuffed-pepper halves on each plate, alongside a generous serving of green beans.

★Dr. V's special tip:

This recipe is perfect for meal prep. If you're cooking for one, prepare the entire batch and refrigerate the extra stuffed peppers in an airtight container. They reheat beautifully and make an easy, nourishing lunch or dinner the next day.

BEER-BRAISED BEEF STEW

There is something deeply comforting about a pot of stew slowly simmering on the stove. Tender beef, vegetables, mushrooms, and a rich broth come together to create a meal that's both hearty and full of flavor. The beer adds remarkable depth of flavor, while the long cooking time transforms simple ingredients into something truly special.
Makes 6 servings.

Ingredients:

- 2 pounds beef chuck roast, cut into 1½-inch cubes
- 2 tablespoons extra-virgin olive oil, plus more if needed
- 1 large yellow onion, diced
- 3 medium carrots, peeled and sliced
- 2 celery stalks, sliced
- 1 orange bell pepper, diced
- 8 ounces white mushrooms, sliced
- 3 garlic cloves, minced
- 2 tablespoons tomato paste
- 1 bottle (12 ounces) beer or gluten-free beer
- 2 cups bone broth or beef broth
- 1 teaspoon balsamic vinegar
- 1 bay leaf
- 1 teaspoon dried thyme
- 1 teaspoon sea salt
- 2 teaspoons Dr. V's Paprika Seasoning (see the recipe at the end of the Dinner Favorites section)
- 2 tablespoons fresh parsley, chopped

Instructions:

1. Pat the beef dry with paper towels.
2. Heat the olive oil in a large pot over medium-high heat.
3. Working in batches, brown the beef on all sides until a deep golden-brown crust forms, about 1–2 minutes per side. Transfer the browned beef to a plate.
4. If the pot appears dry, add a little more olive oil.

5. Reduce the heat to medium and add the onion, carrots, celery, and orange bell pepper. Cook for 5 minutes, stirring occasionally.
6. Add the mushrooms and cook for another 5 minutes, until softened.
7. Add the garlic, tomato paste, and Dr. V's Paprika Seasoning. Cook for 1 minute, stirring constantly.
8. Pour in the beer and use a wooden spoon to scrape up any browned bits from the bottom of the pot.
9. Return the beef and any accumulated juices to the pot.
10. Add the broth, balsamic vinegar, bay leaf, and thyme.
11. Bring to a gentle boil, then reduce the heat to low.
12. Cover and simmer for 2 to 2½ hours, stirring occasionally, until the beef is fork-tender.
13. Remove the bay leaf.
14. Taste and adjust seasoning if needed.
15. Sprinkle with fresh parsley before serving.

★ Dr. V's special tip:

Don't rush the browning step. The deep brown crust that forms on the beef is one of the biggest contributors to the stew's rich flavor.

Like many soups and stews, this recipe tastes even better the next day. Store leftovers in the refrigerator for up to 4 days, or freeze individual portions for an easy future meal.

If you avoid gluten, simply substitute a gluten-free beer. If you prefer not to cook with alcohol, replace the beer with an additional cup of broth.

APPENDIX C

TURMERIC QUINOA WITH SHRIMP

This colorful, protein-rich meal combines tender shrimp, vegetables, and a modest portion of quinoa for a satisfying dish that supports metabolic health without relying on excess carbohydrates. The turmeric gives the quinoa a beautiful golden color while adding an extra layer of flavor. Makes 4 servings.

Ingredients:

For the quinoa and vegetables:

- 1 tablespoon extra-virgin olive oil
- 1 medium onion, finely chopped
- 3 medium carrots, peeled and finely chopped
- 2 celery stalks, thinly sliced
- 1 medium zucchini, diced
- 8 ounces mushrooms, cleaned and sliced
- 1 cup dry quinoa, rinsed thoroughly
- 2 cups bone broth
- 1 teaspoon ground turmeric
- 1 teaspoon sea salt
- ½ teaspoon black pepper

For the shrimp:

- 1½ pounds raw shrimp, peeled and deveined
- 1 tablespoon extra-virgin olive oil
- 1 teaspoon garlic powder
- ½ teaspoon sea salt
- ¼ teaspoon black pepper

Instructions:

Prepare the quinoa and vegetables:

1. Heat 1 tablespoon of olive oil in a large saucepan or deep skillet over medium heat.
2. Add the onion and sauté for 3 to 4 minutes until softened.
3. Add the carrots and celery and continue cooking for 7 minutes, stirring occasionally.

4. Stir in the rinsed quinoa, turmeric, salt, pepper, and mushrooms. Cook for 1 to 2 minutes, stirring frequently.
5. Add the bone broth. Bring the mixture to a gentle boil.
6. Reduce the heat to low, cover, and simmer for 15 minutes.
7. Stir in the zucchini, replace the lid, and continue cooking for 5 to 7 minutes, or until the quinoa is tender and the liquid has been absorbed.
8. Remove from the heat and let stand for 5 minutes before fluffing with a fork.

Prepare the shrimp:

1. While the quinoa cooks, place the shrimp in a bowl and season with garlic powder, salt, and pepper.
2. Heat 1 tablespoon of olive oil in a large skillet over medium-high heat.
3. Add the shrimp in a single layer and cook for 2 to 3 minutes per side, or until pink and opaque. Avoid overcooking.

Serve: Divide the turmeric quinoa and vegetable mixture among plates, top each serving with shrimp, and serve immediately.

★Dr. V's special tip:

If preparing vegetables feels time-consuming, consider investing in a small food processor. It can finely chop vegetables such as onions and carrots in seconds, making healthy cooking much faster and more enjoyable. Many reliable models are available for under $20, making them one of the best kitchen investments for anyone looking to cook more meals at home.

SALMON WITH GOLDEN CAULIFLOWER RICE

Salmon has a reputation for being difficult to cook, but it doesn't have to be. This recipe lets the air fryer do most of the work, producing moist, flaky salmon paired with golden cauliflower rice for a flavorful dinner that's easy enough for any night of the week. Makes 2 servings.

<u>Ingredients:</u>
For the salmon:
- 2 salmon fillets (about 6 ounces each)
- 2 teaspoons butter
- 1 teaspoon dried dill
- Sea salt and black pepper to taste
- Lemon wedges, for serving (optional)

For the golden cauliflower rice:
- 1 medium head cauliflower, grated (or 1 package prepared cauliflower rice)
- 1 tablespoon ghee
- ½ teaspoon ground turmeric
- Sea salt and black pepper to taste

<u>Instructions:</u>
Prepare the salmon:
1. Preheat the air fryer to 400°F.
2. Place the salmon fillets on a parchment paper liner. Top each fillet with 1 teaspoon of butter and season with dill, sea salt, and black pepper.
3. Air fry for 8–10 minutes, or until the salmon flakes easily with a fork. Thicker fillets may require a few additional minutes.

Prepare the golden cauliflower rice:
1. While the salmon cooks, melt the ghee in a large skillet over medium heat.
2. Stir in the turmeric and cook for about 30 seconds, until fragrant.

3. Add the cauliflower rice, season with sea salt and black pepper, cover, and cook for 5–7 minutes, stirring occasionally, until tender.
4. Divide the cauliflower rice between two plates and top with the salmon. Serve with a lemon wedge, if desired.

★ Dr. V's special tip:
Fresh or frozen cauliflower rice both work beautifully in this recipe. If you're starting with a whole head of cauliflower, simply grate it with the large holes of a box grater, but I strongly recommend using a food processor to pulse the florets until they resemble rice.
Don't overcook the salmon. It will continue to cook for a minute or two after it comes out of the air fryer. Removing it just before it's fully done helps keep it moist and tender every time.

APPENDIX C

AIR FRYER CHICKEN WITH ASPARAGUS & MUSHROOMS

Fresh vegetables, juicy chicken, and a handful of seasonings come together to create a colorful meal that's as practical as it is delicious. The air fryer does almost all the work, making this an easy dinner for busy weeknights with very little cleanup. Makes 2 servings.

Ingredients:

For the chicken:

- 2 boneless, skinless chicken breasts
- 1 tablespoon extra-virgin olive oil
- 1 tablespoon Dr. V's Paprika Seasoning (see the recipe at the end of the Dinner Favorites section)
- Sea salt

For the vegetables:

- 4 ounces asparagus, trimmed and cut into 2- to 3-inch pieces
- 4 ounces white mushrooms, sliced
- 2 green onions, sliced
- 2 tablespoons chopped fresh parsley (optional)
- 2 tablespoons extra-virgin olive oil
- Sea salt and black pepper to taste

Instructions:

1. Place the asparagus, mushrooms, green onions, and parsley in a large bowl. Drizzle with the olive oil, season with sea salt and black pepper, and toss well to coat.
2. Arrange the vegetables in a single layer on a parchment paper liner in the air fryer basket. Cook for 8-10 minutes at 400°F, tossing halfway, until tender and lightly browned. Transfer to a serving dish and cover loosely to keep warm.
3. Brush the chicken breasts with the olive oil and season evenly with Dr. V's Paprika Seasoning and some additional salt.
4. Place the chicken on a clean parchment paper liner and air fry for 16-18 minutes, turning halfway, until cooked through.

Cooking time will vary depending on the thickness of the chicken breasts.

5. Serve the chicken alongside the vegetables.

★ Dr. V's special tip:

One of the easiest ways to keep healthy eating sustainable is to let your kitchen appliances do the work. While the air fryer cooks, you're free to prepare the rest of the meal—or simply enjoy a few extra minutes to yourself. If your chicken breasts are especially thick, slice one open to check for doneness before serving.

I recorded a short video of myself preparing this recipe several years ago. It's in Spanish, but cooking is a universal language! If you'd like to see how I chop the vegetables, season everything, and use the air fryer, scan the QR code below for a quick visual demonstration.

CREAMY CHICKEN CURRY WITH ZUCCHINI NOODLES

Warm spices and creamy coconut milk transform everyday ingredients into a flavorful curry. Served over zucchini noodles instead of rice, this curry is a delicious way to enjoy a classic dish while adding another serving of vegetables to your plate.
Makes 4 servings.

Ingredients:
For the curry:

- 2 chicken breasts, cut into bite-sized cubes
- 2 tablespoons ghee, divided
- Sea salt and black pepper to taste
- 1 large yellow onion, finely chopped
- 3 medium carrots, peeled and finely chopped
- 8 ounces white mushrooms, sliced
- 3 garlic cloves, minced
- 1 tablespoon tomato paste
- 1 tablespoon curry powder
- 1 teaspoon ground turmeric
- 1 teaspoon ground ginger (or 1 tablespoon freshly grated ginger)
- 1 (13.5-ounce) can full-fat coconut milk

For the zucchini noodles:

- 2 medium zucchini, spiralized
- 1 teaspoon extra-virgin olive oil
- Sea salt and black pepper to taste

Instructions:

1. Heat 1 tablespoon of the ghee in a large skillet over medium-high heat. Add the chicken, season lightly with sea salt and black pepper, and cook for 3–4 minutes, just until lightly browned on the outside. Transfer to a plate.
2. Add the remaining tablespoon of ghee to the same skillet. Stir in the curry powder, turmeric, and ginger, cooking for about 30 seconds until fragrant.

3. Add the onion and cook for about 3 minutes, until it begins to soften.
4. Add the carrots and mushrooms, cover, and cook for 5–7 minutes, stirring occasionally, until the vegetables begin to soften.
5. Stir in the garlic and tomato paste and cook for 1 minute.
6. Return the chicken and any accumulated juices to the skillet. Pour in the coconut milk, stir well, cover, and simmer for 15–20 minutes, or until the chicken is fully cooked and the vegetables are tender.
7. Meanwhile, heat the olive oil in a separate skillet over medium heat. Add the zucchini noodles, season with sea salt and black pepper, and sauté for 2–3 minutes, just until tender.
8. Divide the zucchini noodles among four plates and spoon the curry over the top.

✯ Dr. V's special tip:

This curry tastes even better the next day as the flavors continue to develop. Store the curry separately from the zucchini noodles or prepare fresh zucchini noodles when reheating for the best texture. If you enjoy a little brightness, serve with a squeeze of fresh lime just before eating.

APPENDIX C

PURA VIDA KETO PIZZA

This pizza has been a family favorite for years. The cauliflower crust is gluten-free, grain-free, and surprisingly sturdy, making it the perfect foundation for plenty of vegetables, quality protein, and flavorful toppings. Makes 2 personal-size pizzas.

Ingredients:
For the crust:
• 3 cups raw cauliflower rice
• 2 large eggs, beaten
• 6 tablespoons almond flour
• 2 teaspoons extra-virgin olive oil
• ½ teaspoon sea salt
• 1 teaspoon Italian seasoning

For the toppings:
• 1 medium tomato, thinly sliced
• 2 cups fresh spinach leaves
• ½ red onion, thinly sliced
• 1 bell pepper, thinly sliced
• 4 ounces mushrooms, sliced
• 4 ounces uncured pepperoni or salami, chopped
• 4 ounces Canadian bacon or minimally processed ham, diced
• 1½ cups shredded mozzarella cheese
• 1 tablespoon dried oregano
• Sea salt and black pepper to taste
• Extra-virgin olive oil for drizzling

Instructions:
Prepare the crust:

1. Preheat the oven to 400°F (200°C). Line two baking sheets or pizza pans with parchment paper.
2. Bring a pot of water to a boil. Add the cauliflower rice and cook for 7 minutes.

3. Drain well and allow it to cool slightly. Transfer the cauliflower to a clean kitchen towel and squeeze out as much moisture as possible; you can also use your hands.
4. Place the cauliflower in a large mixing bowl. Add the eggs, almond flour, olive oil, sea salt, and Italian seasoning. Mix well.
5. Divide the mixture into two equal portions and spread each portion into a thin pizza crust on the prepared parchment paper.
6. Bake for approximately 15 minutes, or until the crusts are firm and lightly golden.

Add the toppings:

7. Remove the crusts from the oven.
8. Arrange the tomato slices evenly over each crust. Top with the spinach, onion, bell pepper, mushrooms, pepperoni, Canadian bacon, and mozzarella cheese.
9. Sprinkle generously with oregano and season lightly with sea salt and black pepper. Finish with a light drizzle of extra-virgin olive oil.
10. Return the pizzas to the oven and bake for an additional 10–15 minutes, or until the cheese is melted and lightly browned.

★Dr. V's special tip:

This is my favorite combination of toppings, but the possibilities are endless. I recorded a video demonstration of this recipe years ago, and it remains one of my favorite cooking memories. The video is in Spanish and captures the joy of sharing good food with family and friends. Scan the QR code below to make this pizza alongside me.

APPENDIX C

DR. V'S PAPRIKA SEASONING

A good seasoning blend can turn everyday ingredients into a flavorful meal in seconds. I keep a jar of this mixture in my pantry and use it regularly on chicken, vegetables, burgers, and more. Make a batch once, and you'll always have an easy way to add flavor without relying on store-bought seasoning mixes. Makes approximately ½ cup.

Ingredients:

- ¼ cup paprika
- 2 teaspoons garlic powder
- 2 teaspoons onion powder
- 2 teaspoons sea salt
- 1 teaspoon black pepper

Instructions:

1. Combine all ingredients in a small bowl.
2. Stir until evenly mixed.
3. Transfer to an airtight glass jar or spice container.
4. Store in a cool, dry place for up to 6 months.

★ Dr. V's special tip:

This blend is meant to be a starting point. Feel free to adjust the proportions to suit your taste. If you enjoy a little heat, add a pinch of cayenne pepper or chili powder.

Treats

DR. V's GIANT AIR FRYER COOKIE

Want a homemade treat without turning on the oven? This giant air fryer cookie comes together in minutes and is made with simple, familiar ingredients. It delivers all the comfort of a freshly baked dessert while providing fiber, healthy fats, and far less sugar than many store-bought alternatives. Perfect for sharing with family or enjoying throughout the week. Makes 4 servings.

Ingredients:

- 1 cup almond flour
- 1 egg
- 2 tablespoons melted butter
- 2 tablespoons allulose
- 1 tablespoon sugar
- 1/4 teaspoon cinnamon
- 1/4 teaspoon baking powder
- 1/4 teaspoon salt
- 1/3 cup dark chocolate chips (80% cacao or higher)
- 1/4 cup chopped pecans

Instructions:

1. In a medium bowl, whisk together the egg, melted butter, allulose, sugar, and cinnamon until well combined.
2. Add almond flour, baking powder, and salt. Stir until a thick dough forms.
3. Fold in the chocolate chips and pecans.
4. Let the dough rest for 3 to 5 minutes to allow the almond flour to absorb moisture.

5. Line the air fryer basket with a round piece of parchment paper. If desired, lightly grease the center with a small amount of coconut oil.
6. Transfer the dough to the parchment paper and shape it into a round cookie about 1/2 inch thick.
7. Air fry at 300°F for 11–13 minutes, or until the edges are lightly golden and the center is set.
8. Allow the cookie to cool for 10–15 minutes before slicing and serving.

Estimated sugar per serving: approximately 9 grams

★Dr. V's special tip:

This recipe makes four servings. If you're not sharing it, cut the cookie into four portions and refrigerate the leftovers. I love enjoying a slice as a dessert after a nutritious meal; it tastes just as delicious chilled the next day.

APPENDIX C

ORANGE CHIA ALMOND MUFFINS

Bright orange zest, warm cinnamon, chia seeds, and sliced almonds come together in these lightly sweetened muffins. They're simple to make and perfect with a morning coffee or as an afternoon treat. Makes approximately 12 muffins.

Ingredients:

- 2 cups almond flour
- ⅓ cup allulose
- 1 teaspoon baking powder
- ¼ teaspoon sea salt
- 1 teaspoon ground cinnamon
- 2 tablespoons chia seeds
- Zest of 1 orange
- ⅓ cup fresh orange juice
- ¼ cup butter, melted
- 3 large eggs
- ⅓ cup sliced almonds, plus more for topping

Instructions:

1. Preheat the oven to 350°F. Grease or line a muffin pan.
2. In a large bowl, combine the almond flour, allulose, baking powder, salt, cinnamon, chia seeds, and sliced almonds.
3. In a separate bowl, whisk together the orange zest, orange juice, melted butter, and eggs.
4. Add the wet ingredients to the dry ingredients and stir well.
5. Divide the batter evenly among the muffin cups, filling each ¾ full. Sprinkle with additional sliced almonds.
6. Bake for 18–22 minutes, or until lightly golden and a toothpick inserted into the center comes out clean.
7. Allow the muffins to cool for 10 minutes before serving.

★ Dr. V's special tip:

Don't skip the orange zest. Most of the orange flavor comes from the zest, not the juice.

APPENDIX C

ENERGY SQUARES

These rich chocolate almond squares come together in just minutes. They don't require baking and store beautifully in the refrigerator. They are perfect when you're looking for a small but satisfying treat.
Makes 6 squares.

Ingredients:

- ¼ cup almond butter
- 2 tablespoons butter, melted
- 2 teaspoons allulose
- 2 tablespoons almond flour
- 2 tablespoons whey protein concentrate
- ¼ teaspoon ground cinnamon
- Pinch of sea salt
- 2 tablespoons unsweetened shredded coconut
- 1 tablespoon pumpkin seeds
- 2 tablespoons dark chocolate chips

Instructions:

1. In a medium bowl, combine the almond butter and melted butter. Stir until smooth.
2. Add the allulose, almond flour, whey protein concentrate, cinnamon, and salt. Stir until well combined.
3. Fold in the shredded coconut, pumpkin seeds, and dark chocolate chips.
4. Line a small container (about 4 × 6 inches) with parchment paper and press the mixture into an even layer.
5. Refrigerate for at least 1 hour, or until firm.
6. Lift out using the parchment paper and cut into 6 squares.

✯ Dr. V's special tip:
These squares become firmer as they chill and taste even better the next day. If you'd like to make a larger batch, simply double the ingredients and use a larger container.

APPENDIX C

AIR FRYER BAKED APPLES

Sometimes the simplest desserts are the most surprising. These warm baked apples are filled with cinnamon, honey, and crunchy nuts, creating a comforting treat with very little effort. Makes 2 servings.

Ingredients:

- 2 Honeycrisp, Pink Lady, or Fuji apples
- 2 teaspoons honey
- 2 tablespoons chopped walnuts or pecans
- ½ teaspoon ground cinnamon
- Pinch of sea salt
- 2 teaspoons butter

Instructions:

1. Wash the apples. Using an apple corer, remove the core from each apple. Cut a small piece from the bottom of the removed core and place it back into the opening to create a plug, leaving a cavity to hold the filling. If you don't have an apple corer, use a small knife and spoon to remove the core while leaving the bottom of the apple intact.
2. Combine the chopped nuts, cinnamon, and sea salt.
3. Fill each apple with half of the nut mixture. Top each with 1 teaspoon of honey and 1 teaspoon of butter.
4. Place the apples in the air fryer basket and cook at 350°F for 18–22 minutes, or until the apples are tender. Begin checking for doneness after 18 minutes, as cooking time may vary with the apples' size and variety. Serve warm.

Oven method:

Place the prepared apples in a small baking dish and bake at 375°F for 30–40 minutes, or until tender.

★ Dr. V's special tip:

Place the apples in the air fryer as you prepare dinner, and by the time you've finished eating, dessert is ready.

PEANUT BUTTER & JELLY UPGRADE

Many people grew up on peanut butter and jelly sandwiches. They're convenient, familiar, and comforting, but traditional versions are often made with highly processed bread and sugary jelly. This upgraded version keeps everything we love about a classic PB&J while using wholesome ingredients and much less sugar. For best results, prepare the strawberry spread in advance and refrigerate it until chilled and thickened. Makes 1 sandwich.

Ingredients:

For the bread:

- 1 tablespoon butter, melted
- 3 tablespoons almond flour
- 1 tablespoon finely chopped pecans
- ½ teaspoon baking powder
- 1 teaspoon allulose
- ¼ teaspoon ground cinnamon
- Pinch of sea salt
- 1 large egg

For the strawberry spread:

- 1 cup frozen strawberries
- 2 tablespoons allulose

For assembly:

- 2 tablespoons natural peanut butter or almond butter

Instructions:

Prepare the bread:

1. In a small 1-cup microwave-safe glass container, combine the melted butter, almond flour, pecans, baking powder, allulose, cinnamon, salt, and egg.
2. Whisk until smooth.
3. Microwave for 90 seconds.
4. Allow the bread to cool for 2–3 minutes.

5. Remove from the container and let cool completely.
6. Slice in half horizontally.

Prepare the strawberry spread:

1. Add the frozen strawberries and allulose to a small saucepan.
2. Cook over medium-low heat for 10–12 minutes, stirring occasionally, until the strawberries are very soft and have released their juices.
3. Allow the mixture to cool slightly.
4. Transfer to a blender or food processor and blend until smooth.
5. Refrigerate until slightly thickened.

Assemble the sandwich:

1. Spread the peanut butter or almond butter on one half of the bread.
2. Spread 1–2 tablespoons of the strawberry spread on the other half.
3. Assemble the sandwich and enjoy.

✭ Dr. V's special tip:

When purchasing peanut butter or almond butter, look for products with the simplest possible ingredient list. Ideally, the only ingredients should be peanuts or almonds, with perhaps a little salt. Avoid products with added sugars, vegetable oils, or unnecessary additives.

The strawberry spread can be stored in the refrigerator for several days and is delicious on yogurt, kefir bowls, cottage cheese, or protein pancakes.

Appendix D

Your Metabolic Restoration Kitchen

One of the questions I'm asked most often is, "What do you always keep at home?" The truth is that healthy eating becomes much easier when your kitchen is stocked with a handful of dependable ingredients and a few basic tools. You don't need a gourmet kitchen or expensive equipment, just a thoughtful collection of staples that make preparing balanced meals feel simple and enjoyable.

Pantry Staples

- Extra-virgin olive oil
- Ghee
- Canned coconut milk
- Bone broth
- Apple cider vinegar
- Balsamic vinegar
- Pure allulose
- Pure liquid stevia
- Sea salt
- Black pepper
- Paprika
- Garlic powder
- Onion powder
- Curry powder
- Turmeric
- Ground cinnamon
- Dried dill
- Almond flour
- Whey protein concentrate
- Collagen peptides
- Chia seeds
- Sesame seeds
- Pumpkin seeds

- Walnuts
- Pecans
- Sliced almonds
- Brazil nuts
- Unsweetened shredded coconut
- Dark chocolate chips
- Canned tuna in extra-virgin olive oil
- Canned sardines in extra-virgin olive oil

Refrigerator Staples

- Eggs
- Butter
- Plain Greek yogurt
- Cottage cheese
- Kefir
- Lemons or limes
- Fresh ginger
- Green onions
- Bell peppers
- Mushrooms
- Carrots
- Zucchini
- Asparagus
- Broccoli
- Avocados
- Garlic
- Fermented vegetables (such as sauerkraut or kimchi)

Freezer Staples

- Frozen berries
- Frozen shrimp
- Frozen cauliflower rice
- Frozen broccoli or mixed vegetables
- Homemade bone broth

- Ice cubes

Kitchen Tools I Use Most Often

- Air fryer
- Blender
- Small food processor
- Spiralizer for zucchini noodles
- Box grater
- Vegetable peeler
- Sharp chef's knife
- Cutting board
- Large skillet
- Large soup pot
- Glass food-storage containers
- Parchment paper liners for the air fryer
- A simple digital scale
- Silicone muffin pan

Appendix E

The Juice Cleanse Reset

What is the JCR?

The Juice Cleanse Reset (JCR) is a structured protocol of vegetable juice and bone broth designed as a short-term therapeutic intervention. It provides an opportunity to temporarily simplify food choices while flooding the body with nutrients derived from vegetables, herbs, roots, and broth.

Even individuals who consider themselves healthy are continuously exposed to ultra-processed foods, environmental toxins, chronic stress, poor sleep, and other factors that place demands on the body's natural detoxification systems. For this reason, the JCR can be repeated annually as an intensive nutritional reset as part of a long-term health strategy.

The JCR is built around a simple principle: when you provide the body with nutrient-dense foods and temporarily remove many of the inputs that contribute to inflammation and metabolic dysfunction, the body can redirect more energy toward repair, recovery, and restoration. This protocol uses what nature provides—real food—in its most concentrated form to support anti-inflammatory and regenerative processes that help the body's cells function at their highest potential.

A primary focus of the JCR is supporting the liver, one of the body's most important metabolic organs. The liver acts as a filtration and processing center, helping eliminate toxins, regulate blood sugar, support digestion, metabolize hormones, and assist with the absorption and utilization of many nutrients. Because of its central role in health, supporting liver function can have far-reaching effects throughout the body.

Many individuals report improvements in energy, digestion, bloating, skin health, mental clarity, and overall well-being during or after completing the JCR. Individual experiences vary, but the goal is to provide the body with a temporary period of deep nutritional support and create an opportunity for meaningful change.

APPENDIX E

This protocol was inspired in part by the Spanish-language booklet *#YoPuedo* by Dra. Coco March, as well as the documentary *Fat, Sick & Nearly Dead* by Joe Cross, both of which helped shape the development of the JCR.

If you choose to complete this program, please read this appendix in its entirety before beginning. If you are pregnant, breastfeeding, underweight, have a history of an eating disorder, have diabetes, take medications that affect blood sugar or blood pressure, have kidney disease, have significant medical conditions, or are unsure whether this protocol is appropriate for you, consult your healthcare provider before starting.

Choosing a Juicer

Before beginning the JCR, make sure you have everything you need. The most important piece of equipment is a juicer. A blender cannot be used as a substitute because it does not separate the juice from the pulp. During the JCR, the goal is to consume vegetable juice without the fiber. By temporarily removing most of the fiber from the vegetables, the digestive system has less work to do, allowing nutrients to be absorbed quickly while simplifying the digestive process.

Green juices provide a concentrated source of vitamins, minerals, phytonutrients, and plant compounds derived from vegetables, herbs, roots, and small amounts of fruit.

There are two primary types of juicers. Masticating juicers, also known as cold-press juicers, operate at a slower speed and are generally thought to preserve more nutrients during juicing. They tend to perform especially well with leafy greens, but are often more expensive and require more time to use. Examples include the Ninja Cold-Press Juicer Pro, Omega Series, and Aucma Slow Masticating Juicer.

Centrifugal juicers operate at a much higher speed and are typically faster and more affordable. While they may not extract as much juice from leafy vegetables, they can still produce excellent results and are often a practical option. Examples include the Breville Juice Fountain series and the Mueller Ultra Power Juicer.

Either type of juicer can be used successfully. The best juicer is the one that fits your budget, lifestyle, and likelihood of consistent use. The brands listed above are provided only as examples and do not constitute an endorsement.

What to Expect During the First Few Days

As your body adapts to a very different nutritional pattern, it is not unusual to experience temporary symptoms during the first several days of the JCR. While some individuals feel energized almost immediately, others notice a brief adjustment period before they begin feeling better.

One of the most common changes is increased urination. This occurs because reducing carbohydrates and lowering insulin levels often allows the body to release excess fluid that has been retained for months or even years. As this fluid is eliminated, you might notice mild changes in energy levels, blood pressure, or overall well-being.

Because every person is different, it is impossible to predict exactly how you will respond. Some people experience very few symptoms, while others notice several. Common temporary symptoms may include headaches, fatigue, weakness, brain fog, irritability, cravings, nausea, bloating, skin changes, sleep disturbances, diarrhea, or constipation.

Many people are surprised by these symptoms and mistakenly assume they are getting sick. In most cases, these reactions are temporary and reflect the body's adaptation to a new nutritional environment. Staying well hydrated, consuming adequate bone broth, prioritizing rest, and trusting the process can make the transition more comfortable.

It is also important to understand that bowel movements often become less frequent during the Juicing Phase. Because very little fiber is consumed, less material moves through the digestive tract. This is expected and does not necessarily indicate a problem.

Most temporary symptoms improve within a few days as the body adjusts. However, if you experience severe symptoms, worsening symptoms, or anything that concerns you, discontinue the protocol and consult your healthcare provider.

APPENDIX E

Phase 1: The Juice Reset

Phase 1 lasts twenty-one days. During this phase, you will consume only vegetable juices, organic chicken bone broth, water, herbal teas, and optional coffee.

There is no need to restrict how much juice, broth, water, or tea you consume. You should not spend the day feeling excessively hungry or thirsty. Listen to your body's signals and drink as needed.

Most people consume approximately 2 liters (about ½ gallon) of vegetable juice and at least 1 liter of organic chicken bone broth per day. Fresh juice is ideal, but it is usually more practical to juice once daily or every other day. Store juice and broth in tightly sealed glass containers and refrigerate until ready to use. I find it helpful to store both in 16-ounce individual servings that are ready to grab and go.

Hunger and cravings are common early in the program. These sensations typically become less intense as the body adapts to a different eating pattern. A helpful strategy is to drink something whenever hunger appears. This means consuming juice, broth, tea, or water approximately every two hours while awake.

Organic chicken bone broth plays an important role during this phase. It provides minerals, amino acids, collagen, and warmth while helping many people feel more satisfied throughout the day. You may drink as much broth as desired. Homemade broth is an excellent option, though high-quality organic store-bought chicken bone broth can also work well. Feel free to season it with natural herbs, spices, or mineral salt to taste. Avoid using bouillon cubes as a substitute.

Daily Guidelines

It is highly recommended to begin the day with a small glass of water containing one teaspoon of organic apple cider vinegar (ACV) with the mother. If desired, you may add a small amount of extra-virgin olive oil to make it easier to tolerate. Apple cider vinegar may help support healthy blood sugar regulation, digestion, and metabolic function.

Coffee is permitted during the JCR. If you prefer a sweetener, choose allulose, stevia, or monk fruit in their purest forms. A very small amount of half-and-half or milk is acceptable, but avoid flavored creamers and heavily processed coffee additives. You can also add pure vanilla extract and/or MCT oil.

Hydration is essential throughout the JCR. Drink plenty of purified water and consider using mineral-rich salt, such as Himalayan salt, in your broth to help support electrolyte balance.

A Typical Day During Phase 1

6:30 AM: 1 small glass of water with one tsp of ACV with the mother
7:00 AM: Coffee or tea
8:00 AM: Juice (500 ml or 16 oz)
10:00 AM: Organic chicken bone broth (500 ml or 16 oz)
12:00 PM: Juice (500 ml or 16 oz)
2:00 PM: Organic chicken bone broth (500 ml or 16 oz)
4:00 PM: Juice (500 ml or 16 oz)
6:00 PM: Organic chicken bone broth (500 ml or 16 oz)
8:00 PM: Juice (500 ml) or organic chicken bone broth (500ml)

There is no need to follow a rigid schedule. The goal is to remain hydrated, nourished, and comfortable while avoiding solid food during Phase 1.

Chicken Bone Broth Recipe

- 1.5 to 2 pounds of organic chicken feet (can be found at stores such as Whole Foods)
- 1 pound of celery
- 1 pound of carrots
- 1 whole garlic head cut right in the middle
- 1 bell pepper or chili
- 2 tomatoes, diced or grated
- 1 big onion
- Salt and pepper

Put everything in a big pot with 1.5 to 2 gallons of water. Bring it to a boil and then gently simmer for about 12-15 hours. When it cools down, strain it and bottle it in 500 ml mason jars, so it is ready to go in individual servings.

Ginger and Cinnamon Tea

- 2 cinnamon sticks
- 1-piece fresh ginger
- Water
- Boil for 10–15 minutes.

Juice Preparation

The recipes that follow are intended as examples and can be modified to suit preferences and availability. The Basic Green Juice can be used as your foundation throughout the entire program. For those who prefer more variety, I have also included seven juice recipes.

When juicing citrus fruits, you may include a small amount of the peel if the fruit is organic. However, use caution, as the peel can create a strong, unpleasant flavor.

Always be mindful of food allergies or sensitivities and avoid any ingredient that may cause a reaction. Do not add water to your juices. Finally, remember that vegetables should make up the vast majority of your juice. The less fruit you add, the better.

Basic Green Juice (Makes about 2 liters)

Carrots	1,000 grams	35 oz
Celery	500 grams	18 oz
Cucumbers	700 grams	24 oz
Green leafy vegetables	250 grams	9 oz
Ginger	20 grams	1 oz
Turmeric	25 grams	1 oz
Green apple	1 unit	1 unit
Lemon	1 unit, peeled	1 unit, peeled
Other vegetables or fruits of your choice	500 grams	18 oz

APPENDIX E

Juice Recipes for 7 days

Green Monster	**Purple Love**
2 handfuls of baby spinach (8 oz) Whole Kale leaves A bunch of parsley or cilantro Ginger and turmeric roots Carrots Celery Cucumbers 1 green bell pepper 1 zucchini Broccoli 1 green apple 1 lemon 2 oranges	2 handfuls of green leafy vegetables (8 oz) Ginger and turmeric roots 1 grapefruit Carrots 1 apple 1 orange 1 lemon 1 red bell pepper 1 cucumber Celery Purple cabbage Radish with the tops 1 eggplant
Minty Energy	**V-9**
2 handfuls of green leafy vegetables (8 oz) Ginger and turmeric roots A bunch of fresh mint leaves 1 grapefruit Carrots 1 orange 1 lemon Celery Cauliflower 1 cucumber Jicama Green cabbage	2 handfuls of green leafy vegetables (8 oz) Parsley Cilantro Ginger and turmeric roots Carrots 2 tomatoes 1 green bell pepper 1 Romaine lettuce head Celery Cucumber Green grapes

Tropical Sunshine One Romaine lettuce head Ginger and turmeric roots 1 slice of Pineapple Carrots Celery 2 Kiwi Papaya Sweet potatoes Watermelon	**Citrus Delight** Swiss chard Ginger and turmeric roots Carrots Cucumbers Limes Lemons Oranges 2 grapefruit
Red Splendor Beets with tops Ginger and turmeric roots Strawberries Cantaloupe Celery Cucumber Lemons 1 orange	*Continue rotating these recipes, using the Basic Green Juice, or creating your own combinations for the remainder of Phase 1*

Phase 2: The Transition Phase

Congratulations. By completing Phase 1, you have already accomplished the most challenging part of the JCR. Twenty-one days is a significant commitment, and you should be proud of what you have achieved.

Phase 2 lasts seven days and serves as a bridge between the Juice Reset and a sustainable, long-term way of eating, such as the 28-Day Metabolic Restoration program (28-MR). During this phase, you will begin reintroducing solid foods while continuing many of the habits established during Phase 1.

APPENDIX E

The foods introduced during Phase 2 are nutrient-dense, minimally processed, and designed to support your transition back to solid food. It is important to reintroduce food gradually. After three weeks without solid food, your digestive system may need time to adapt. Eat slowly, and pay attention to hunger and fullness cues.

Phase 2 Eating Plan

Each day, continue consuming:

- 32 ounces (1 liter) of vegetable juice
- Organic chicken bone broth as desired
- Ginger-cinnamon tea as desired
- Plenty of filtered water

In addition, add:

- One organic apple per day
- One large salad with protein
- Three teaspoons of chia seeds daily
- One high-quality protein shake

Chia seeds can be added to your salad, mixed into your shake, stirred into juice, or consumed with water. Protein options may include tuna, salmon, chicken, or turkey. You might choose to postpone red meat until digestion has fully adjusted to eating solid food again.

<u>Large Salad Recipe</u>

- A generous serving of leafy greens (spinach, lettuce, spring mix)
- Tomato
- Onion
- Carrot
- Cucumber
- Bell pepper
- ½ avocado
- Mineral salt and pepper
- Balsamic vinegar
- Extra-virgin olive oil or avocado oil
- Tuna, salmon, chicken, or turkey

APPENDIX E

Protein Shake Recipe

- 8–12 ounces unsweetened non-dairy milk, such as almond or coconut milk
- One serving of a high-quality protein powder
- 2 tablespoons coconut oil or ½ avocado
- Ice, optional

At this point, you are ready to transition into the principles of Metabolic Restoration described in Chapter 10. The JCR was designed to be a reset, not a destination. The habits you build moving forward will ultimately have the greatest impact on your long-term health

Appendix F

The Books That Helped Shape Me

These are some of the books that deeply influenced the way I think about metabolism, prevention, women's health, longevity, the nervous system, brain health, and the connection between lifestyle and healing.

- **The Diabetes Code** — by Jason Fung. Helped me understand insulin resistance and type 2 diabetes through a completely different lens, focused on root causes rather than symptom management.

- **Nature Wants Us to Be Fat** — by Richard J. Johnson. Opened my eyes to the evolutionary and biochemical mechanisms that drive fat storage and modern metabolic disease.

- **The Obesity Code** — by Jason Fung. Reinforced the powerful role of hormones, especially insulin, in weight regulation and metabolic health.

- **Why We Get Sick** — by Benjamin Bikman. Simplified the concept that insulin resistance sits at the center of many chronic diseases.

- **Syndrome X** — by Jack Challem and Burton Berkson. Helped connect metabolic dysfunction to a broad spectrum of chronic illness.

- **Metabolical** — by Robert Lustig. Deepened my understanding of processed food, modern nutrition, and the collision between industry and health.

APPENDIX F

- **Keto Diet** — by Josh Axe. Offered practical insight into ketogenic nutrition and metabolic flexibility in an approachable way.

- **Healing PCOS** — by Amy Medling. Highlighted how lifestyle, nutrition, and hormone balance can profoundly impact women with PCOS.

- **Glucose Revolution** — by Jessie Inchauspé. Made blood sugar science incredibly practical and easy to apply in everyday life.

- **Real Food for Pregnancy** — by Lily Nichols. Completely changed the way I think about prenatal nutrition and evidence-based nourishment during pregnancy.

- **The Continuous Glucose Monitor Revolution** — by Paul Kolodzik. Strengthened my appreciation for continuous glucose monitoring as a tool for prevention and self-awareness.

- **Hashimoto's Protocol** — by Izabella Wentz. Expanded my understanding of autoimmune thyroid disease and the importance of personalized lifestyle interventions.

- **Fast Like a Girl** — by Mindy Pelz. Inspired me to think about fasting through the unique physiology and hormonal rhythms of women.

- **Brain Energy** — by Christopher Palmer. Profoundly impacted the way I see the connection between metabolism, mitochondrial health, and mental health.

- **Outlive** — by Peter Attia. Encouraged a proactive, prevention-centered approach to longevity and modern medicine.

APPENDIX F

- **Brain Maker** — by David Perlmutter. Helped me appreciate the powerful relationship between the gut microbiome and brain health.

- **Brain Food** — by Lisa Mosconi. Deepened my understanding of how nutrition uniquely impacts the female brain across the lifespan.

- **Lifespan** — by David Sinclair. Sparked curiosity about aging biology and the future possibilities of longevity science.

- **Longevity Guidebook** — by Peter Diamandis. Reinforced the idea that technology, prevention, and lifestyle can radically reshape the future of healthspan.

- **Why We Sleep** — by Matthew Walker. Completely transformed the way I view sleep, helping me understand that sleep is one of the foundational pillars of health.

- **Breath** — by James Nestor. Deepened my appreciation for the profound impact that breathing patterns can have on stress, focus, nervous system regulation, and overall well-being.

- **El milagro metabólico** — by Carlos Jaramillo. Offered a powerful and accessible perspective on metabolic health for the Spanish-speaking community.

References

[1] Chen J, Fu D, Ma T, Chen M, Wang X, Yi J. *Global burden of metabolic disorders among women of child-bearing age, 1990–2021: a population-based study.* BMC Women's Health. 2025;25:207. doi:10.1186/s12905-025-03749-5.

[2] Jun D, Knowles K, Fazzino TL. *Examination of hyper-palatable foods and their nutrient characteristics using globally crowdsourced data.* PLOS ONE. 2025;20(6):e0325479. doi:10.1371/journal.pone.0325479.

[3] Story M, French S. *Food advertising and marketing directed at children and adolescents in the US.* International Journal of Behavioral Nutrition and Physical Activity. 2004;1:3. doi:10.1186/1479-5868-1-3.

[4] Wang Y, Qi T, Wu X, et al. *Ultra-processed foods, biological ageing, and all-cause mortality risk: a prospective cohort study using 172,225 participants from UK Biobank.* GeroScience. 2025;47(5):6599–6612.

[5] Ranabir S, Reetu K. Stress and hormones. Indian J Endocrinol Metab. 2011;15(1):18-22. doi:10.4103/2230-8210.77573

[6] Monteiro CA, Cannon G. Yes, Food Portion Sizes and People Have Become Bigger and Bigger. What Is to Be Done?. *Am J Public Health.* 2021;111(12):2091-2093. doi:10.2105/AJPH.2021.306547

[7] Taegtmeyer H, Beauloye C, Harmancey R, Hue L. Comment on Nolan et al. Insulin Resistance as a Physiological Defense Against Metabolic Stress: Implications for the Management of Subsets of Type 2 Diabetes. Diabetes 2015;64:673-686. *Diabetes*. 2015;64(10):e37. doi:10.2337/db15-0655

[8] Frates B. The Evolving State of Nutrition Education. *Am J Lifestyle Med.* 2023;17(6):759-761. Published 2023 Jul 7. doi:10.1177/15598276231187582

[9] Krishnan S, Sytsma T, Wischmeyer PE. *Addressing the urgent need for clinical nutrition education in postgraduate medical training: New programs and credentialing.* Journal of the Academy of Nutrition and Dietetics. 2024. doi:10.1016/j.jadnut.2024.100321.

[10] Waldman SA, Terzic A. Health Care Evolves From Reactive to Proactive. *Clin Pharmacol Ther.* 2019;105(1):10-13. doi:10.1002/cpt.1295

[11] Micha R, Mozaffarian D. Trans fatty acids: effects on metabolic syndrome, heart disease and diabetes. *Nat Rev Endocrinol.* 2009;5(6):335-344. doi:10.1038/nrendo.2009.79

[12] Lustig RH. *Metabolical: The Lure and the Lies of Processed Food, Nutrition, and Modern Medicine.* New York, NY: Harper Wave; 2021.

[13] Foley PJ. Effect of low carbohydrate diets on insulin resistance and the metabolic syndrome. *Curr Opin Endocrinol Diabetes Obes.* 2021;28(5):463-468. doi:10.1097/MED.0000000000000065

[14] Lonnie M, Hooker E, Brunstrom JM, et al. *Protein for Life: Review of Optimal Protein Intake, Sustainable Dietary Sources and the Effect on Appetite in Ageing Adults.* Nutrients. 2018;10(3):360. doi:10.3390/nu10030360

[15] Johnson RJ, Sánchez-Lozada LG, Andrews P, Lanaspa MA. Perspective: A Historical and Scientific Perspective of Sugar and Its Relation with Obesity and Diabetes. *Adv Nutr.* 2017;8(3):412-422. Published 2017 May 15. doi:10.3945/an.116.014654

[16] World Health Organization. *WHO calls on countries to reduce sugars intake among adults and children.* Published March 4, 2015. Accessed June 3, 2026. https://www.who.int/news/item/04-03-2015-who-calls-on-countries-to-reduce-sugars-intake-among-adults-and-children

[17] Avner S, Robbins T. A Scoping Review of Glucose Spikes in People Without Diabetes: Comparing Insights from Grey Literature and Medical Research. *Clin Med Insights Endocrinol Diabetes*. 2025;18:11795514251381409. Published 2025 Oct 25. doi:10.1177/11795514251381409

[18] Avena NM, Rada P, Hoebel BG. Evidence for sugar addiction: behavioral and neurochemical effects of intermittent, excessive sugar intake. *Neurosci Biobehav Rev*. 2008;32(1):20-39. doi:10.1016/j.neubiorev.2007.04.019

[19] Coccurello R. Disrupting the Gut-Brain Axis: How Artificial Sweeteners Rewire Microbiota and Reward Pathways. *Int J Mol Sci*. 2025;26(20):10220. Published 2025 Oct 21. doi:10.3390/ijms262010220

[20] Wise PM, Nattress L, Flammer LJ, Beauchamp GK. Reduced dietary intake of simple sugars alters perceived sweet taste intensity but not perceived pleasantness. *Am J Clin Nutr*. 2016;103(1):50-60. doi:10.3945/ajcn.115.112300

[21] Brisendine MH, Drake JC. Integrative physiology of skeletal muscle for maintaining cognitive health. J Physiol. 2026;604:2448-2457. doi:10.1113/JP286748

[22] Currier BS, Ferraro ZM, Mazzulla M, et al. *Resistance training prescription for muscle strength and hypertrophy in healthy adults: a systematic review and Bayesian network meta-analysis*. British Journal of Sports Medicine. 2023;57(18):1211–1220.

[23] Lin D, Zhang L, Huang C, Shao W. Skeletal muscle metabolism in health and disease: Mechanisms, interventions, and clinical perspectives. *iScience*. 2026;29(3):115024. Published 2026 Feb 14. doi:10.1016/j.isci.2026.115024

[24] Rantanen T, Masaki K, He Q, Ross GW, Willcox BJ, White L. Midlife muscle strength and human longevity up to age 100 years: a 44-year prospective study among a decedent cohort. *Age (Dordr)*. 2012;34(3):563-570. doi:10.1007/s11357-011-9256-y

[25] Andaloro S, Cacciatore S, Risoli A, et al. Hip Fracture as a Systemic Disease in Older Adults: A Narrative Review on Multisystem Implications and Management. *Med Sci (Basel)*. 2025;13(3):89. Published 2025 Jul 11. doi:10.3390/medsci13030089

[26] Fragala MS, Cadore EL, Dorgo S, et al. Resistance Training for Older Adults: Position Statement From the National Strength and Conditioning Association. *J Strength Cond Res*. 2019;33(8):2019-2052. doi:10.1519/JSC.0000000000003230

[27] Chuah TY, Lim CY, Tan RZ, et al. Functional Reference Limits: Describing Physiological Relationships and Determination of Physiological Limits for Enhanced Interpretation of Laboratory Results. *Ann Lab Med*. 2023;43(5):408-417. doi:10.3343/alm.2023.43.5.408

[28] Kasuga M. Insulin resistance and pancreatic beta cell failure. *J Clin Invest*. 2006;116(7):1756-1760. doi:10.1172/JCI29189

[29] Sagesaka H, Sato Y, Someya Y, et al. Type 2 Diabetes: When Does It Start?. *J Endocr Soc*. 2018;2(5):476-484. Published 2018 Apr 18. doi:10.1210/js.2018-00071

[30] Thomas DD, Corkey BE, Istfan NW, Apovian CM. Hyperinsulinemia: An Early Indicator of Metabolic

Dysfunction. *J Endocr Soc*. 2019;3(9):1727-1747. Published 2019 Jul 24. doi:10.1210/js.2019-00065

[31] Almohtasib Y, Fancher AJ, Sawalha K. Emerging Trends in Atherosclerosis: Time to Address Atherosclerosis From a Younger Age. *Cureus*. 2024;16(3):e56635. Published 2024 Mar 21. doi:10.7759/cureus.56635

[32] Dhondge RH, Agrawal S, Patil R, Kadu A, Kothari M. A Comprehensive Review of Metabolic Syndrome and Its Role in Cardiovascular Disease and Type 2 Diabetes Mellitus: Mechanisms, Risk Factors, and Management. *Cureus*. 2024;16(8):e67428. Published 2024 Aug 21. doi:10.7759/cureus.67428

[33] Walker MP, Stickgold R. Sleep, memory, and plasticity. *Annu Rev Psychol*. 2006;57:139-166. doi:10.1146/annurev.psych.56.091103.070307

[34] Walker MP. *Why We Sleep: Unlocking the Power of Sleep and Dreams*. New York, NY: Scribner; 2017.

[35] Watson NF, Badr MS, Belenky G, et al. Recommended Amount of Sleep for a Healthy Adult: A Joint Consensus Statement of the American Academy of Sleep Medicine and Sleep Research Society. *Sleep*. 2015;38(6):843-844. Published 2015 Jun 1. doi:10.5665/sleep.4716

[36] Spira AP, Chen-Edinboro LP, Wu MN, Yaffe K. Impact of sleep on the risk of cognitive decline and dementia. *Curr Opin Psychiatry*.2014;27(6):478-483. doi:10.1097/YCO.0000000000000106

[37] Onyegbule CJ, Muoghalu CG, Ofoegbu CC, Ezeorah F. The Impact of Poor Sleep Quality on Cardiovascular Risk Factors and

Quality of Life. *Cureus*. 2025;17(1):e77397. Published 2025 Jan 13. doi:10.7759/cureus.77397

[38] Nestor J. *Breath: The New Science of a Lost Art.* New York, NY: Riverhead Books; 2020.

[39] Encarnação T, Pais AA, Campos MG, Burrows HD. Endocrine disrupting chemicals: Impact on human health, wildlife and the environment. *Sci Prog*. 2019;102(1):3-42. doi:10.1177/0036850419826802

[40] Díaz-Galiano FJ, Gómez-Ramos MJ, Beraza I, Murcia-Morales M, Fernández-Alba AR. Cooking food in microwavable plastic containers: in situ formation of a new chemical substance and increased migration of polypropylene polymers. *Food Chem*. 2023;417:135852. doi:10.1016/j.foodchem.2023.135852

[41] Adil N, Ashraf K, Munir M, Mohiuddin M, Abbasi A, Riaz U, Aslam A, Marey SA, Hatamleh AA, Zaman Qu. Pesticides, Heavy Metals and Plasticizers: Contamination and Risk Assessment of Drinking-Water Quality. *Sustainability*. 2023; 15(17):13263. doi.org/10.3390/su151713263

[42] Nihart AJ, Garcia MA, El Hayek E, et al. Bioaccumulation of microplastics in decedent human brains. *Nat Med*. 2025;31(4):1114-1119. doi:10.1038/s41591-024-03453-1

[43] Potera C. Scented products emit a bouquet of VOCs. *Environ Health Perspect*. 2011;119(1):A16. doi:10.1289/ehp.119-a16

[44] Schmidt S. Acknowledging Receipts? New Evidence for Dermal Absorption of Bisphenols. *Environ Health Perspect*. 2020;128(3):34003. doi:10.1289/EHP6249

[45] Goodman MJ. The “Natural” vs. “Natural Flavors” Conflict in Food Labeling: A Regulatory Viewpoint. *Food Drug Law J*. 2017;72(1):78-102.

[46] Arnold LE, Lofthouse N, Hurt E. Artificial food colors and attention-deficit/hyperactivity symptoms: conclusions to dye for. *Neurotherapeutics*. 2012;9(3):599-609. doi:10.1007/s13311-012-0133-x

[47] Naimi S, Viennois E, Gewirtz AT, Chassaing B. Direct impact of commonly used dietary emulsifiers on human gut microbiota. *Microbiome*. 2021;9(1):66. Published 2021 Mar 22. doi:10.1186/s40168-020-00996-6

[48] Rondinella D, Raoul PC, Valeriani E, et al. The Detrimental Impact of Ultra-Processed Foods on the Human Gut Microbiome and Gut Barrier. *Nutrients*. 2025;17(5):859. Published 2025 Feb 28. doi:10.3390/nu17050859

[49] Lyon, G. (2024). *Forever Strong Playbook*. Institute for Muscle-Centric Medicine.

[50] Arias E, Xu J. *United States Life Tables, 2018*. National Vital Statistics Reports. 2020;69(12):1-45. Hyattsville, MD: National Center for Health Statistics.

[51] Cook G. Quieting "Food Noise": How GLP-1s and Mindfulness Rewire the Default Mode Network (DMN) and Reward Circuits. *Cureus*. 2026;18(1):e100818. Published 2026 Jan 5. doi:10.7759/cureus.100818

[52] Kreouzi M, Theodorakis N, Constantinou C. Lessons Learned From Blue Zones, Lifestyle Medicine Pillars and Beyond: An Update on the Contributions of Behavior and Genetics to Wellbeing and Longevity. *Am J Lifestyle Med*. 2022;18(6):750-765. Published 2022 Aug 20. doi:10.1177/15598276221118494

[53] United States Census Bureau. *QuickFacts: Las Cruces city, New Mexico*. U.S. Census Bureau. Accessed June 3, 2026.

https://www.census.gov/quickfacts/fact/table/lascrucescitynewmexico/PST045224

[54] Michael A. Singer, *The Untethered Soul: The Journey Beyond Yourself* (Oakland, CA: New Harbinger Publications, 2007). If I can hear that voice, who is the one listening?

www.ingramcontent.com/pod-product-compliance
Lightning Source LLC
LaVergne TN
LVHW090400210926
848480LV00002B/401
9798996845002